S0-ARN-246

Genetics in Practice

Property of Library
Cape Fear Community College
Wilmington, NC

Genetics in Practice

A clinical approach for healthcare practitioners

JO HAYDON

Senior Genetic Counsellor and Nurse Specialist in Genetics Education
Centre for Education in Medical Genetics
West Midlands Regional Clinical Genetics Service

John Wiley & Sons, Ltd

Copyright © 2007   John Wiley & Sons Ltd, The Atrium, Southern Gate, Chichester,
West Sussex PO19 8SQ, England

Telephone   (+44) 1243 779777

Email (for orders and customer service enquiries): cs-books@wiley.co.uk
Visit our Home Page on www.wiley.com

All Rights Reserved. No part of this publication may be reproduced, stored in a retrieval system or transmitted in any
form or by any means, electronic, mechanical, photocopying, recording, scanning or otherwise, except under the
terms of the Copyright, Designs and Patents Act 1988 or under the terms of a licence issued by the Copyright
Licensing Agency Ltd, 90 Tottenham Court Road, London W1T 4LP, UK, without the permission in writing of the
Publisher. Requests to the Publisher should be addressed to the Permissions Department, John Wiley & Sons Ltd, The
Atrium, Southern Gate, Chichester, West Sussex PO19 8SQ, England, or emailed to permreq@wiley.co.uk, or faxed
to (+44) 1243 770620.

Designations used by companies to distinguish their products are often claimed as trademarks. All brand names and
product names used in this book are trade names, service marks, trademarks or registered trademarks of their
respective owners. The Publisher is not associated with any product or vendor mentioned in this book.

This publication is designed to provide accurate and authoritative information in regard to the subject matter covered.
It is sold on the understanding that the Publisher is not engaged in rendering professional services. If professional
advice or other expert assistance is required, the services of a competent professional should be sought.

Other Wiley Editorial Offices

John Wiley & Sons Inc., 111 River Street, Hoboken, NJ 07030, USA

Jossey-Bass, 989 Market Street, San Francisco, CA 94103-1741, USA

Wiley-VCH Verlag GmbH, Boschstr. 12, D-69469 Weinheim, Germany

John Wiley & Sons Australia Ltd, 42 McDougall Street, Milton, Queensland 4064, Australia

John Wiley & Sons (Asia) Pte Ltd, 2 Clementi Loop #02-01, Jin Xing Distripark, Singapore 129809

John Wiley & Sons Canada Ltd, 6045 Freemont Blvd, Mississauga, ONT, L5R 4J3, Canada

Wiley also publishes its books in a variety of electronic formats. Some content that appears in print may not be
available in electronic books.

Anniversary Logo Design: Richard J. Pacifico

Library of Congress Cataloging-in-Publication Data

Haydon, Jo.
   Genetics in practice : a clinical approach for healthcare practitioners / Jo Haydon.
      p. ; cm.
   Includes index
   ISBN 978-1-86156-464-1 (pbk. : alk. paper)
   1. Medical genetics.   2. Genetic disorders—Diagnosis.   3. Genetic counseling.   4. Nursing.
   I. Title.   [DNLM: 1. Genetics, Medical—methods—Nurses' Instruction.   2. Genetic Diseases,
   Inborn—diagnosis—Nurses' Instruction.   3. Genetic Predisposition to Disease—Nurses' Instruction.
   4. Genetic Services—Nurses' Instruction.   QZ 50 H416g 2007]
   RB155.H39 2007
   616′.042—dc22

                                                                                              2007026600

British Library Cataloguing in Publication Data

A catalogue record for this book is available from the British Library

ISBN: 978-1-86156-464-1

Typeset in 10/12pt Times by Integra Software Services Pvt. Ltd, Pondicherry, India
Printed and bound in Great Britain by TJ International, Padstow, UK.
This book is printed on acid-free paper responsibly manufactured from sustainable forestry in which
at least two trees are planted for each one used for paper production.

Contents

List of Contributors

Amanda Barry
Registered Genetic Counsellor, Clinical Genetics Unit, West Midlands Regional Clinical Genetics Service, Birmingham Women's Hospital; amanda.barry@bwhct.nhs.uk

Lucy Burgess
Cancer Genetic Counsellor, Clinical Genetics Unit, West Midlands Regional Clinical Genetics Service, Birmingham Women's Hospital; lucy.burgess@bwhct.nhs.uk

Professor Peter Farndon
Professor of Clinical Genetics and Consultant Geneticist, Clinical Genetics Unit, West Midlands Regional Clinical Genetics Service, Birmingham Women's Hospital; peter.farndon@bwhct.nhs.uk

Eileen Roberts
Consultant Scientist in Cytogenetics, Bristol Genetics Laboratory, Southmead Hospital, Bristol

Dr Sarah Warburton
National Training Co-ordinator for Clinical Molecular Genetics, National Genetics Education and Development Centre, Birmingham Women's Hospital; sarah.warburton@bwhct.nhs.uk

Tessa Webb
Lecturer in Medical Genetics, Birmingham University; t.webb@bham.ac.uk

Preface

Human genetics and its clinical application is a fast developing sphere impinging on all areas of healthcare professionals' practice. It is hoped that this book will provide a comprehensive introduction to present-day genetic services, including the role of the genetic counsellor.

The aim of this book is to raise healthcare professionals' awareness of how genetics impacts on all areas of healthcare and of the effect of a genetic diagnosis on the individual and their family. The clinical genetics service provides information for families (often including a diagnosis) and aims to support individuals and their families and to enable them to make informed choices relevant to their genetic situation. In facilitating decision making it is vital that practitioners remain supportive and non-directive. It is therefore important for individuals and families to understand the relevant mechanisms of inheritance, the possible tests available and the options that are open to them.

During my practice as a genetic counsellor I have experienced the rapid expansion of knowledge in this field and the consequent increased needs of families for support in understanding and facilitating choices available to them. It is an exciting and challenging area of healthcare and one that now affects healthcare professionals in all areas of clinical practice.

This book aims to provide the healthcare professional with basic knowledge and awareness of genetics and thus to aid understanding of the needs of their patients.

Introduction

At a time of rapid developments in the field of human genetics, this book aims to dispel some of the mystique surrounding the subject, in order to enable healthcare professionals to recognise its relevance in their everyday clinical practice. It provides a basic text for healthcare professionals, covering the main issues that an individual and their family are confronted with when a genetic diagnosis is made. It is not intended to provide comprehensive details of all, or even the commonest, genetic disorders. Such books are available elsewhere, and these may not address the healthcare professional's role with affected families.

When a genetic diagnosis is made, individuals and their families need support in coming to terms with both the diagnosis and the prognosis. They also need help to appreciate the implications for their current or future offspring and other members of the extended family. Support must also be available to members of the extended family whose future options may be affected by the medical implications of the diagnosis. When such a diagnosis is made by the clinical genetics service, genetic counsellors play a major role in providing the initial support but healthcare professionals in other relevant specialties will be involved in the continuing support of the individual/family. The same condition can have differing implications for different families and even for different individuals within the same family. It is therefore important that family-centred, not diagnosis-led, care is provided for these individuals and their families. This concept has governed the way this book is written. It is factual in nature and uses real-life case studies to demonstrate the application of theoretical principles to clinical practice. The case studies cover the whole life span from prenatal diagnosis, through childhood and adult-onset disorders.

The first chapter of the book introduces the reader to the history of genetics and the developments that have occurred to bring us to present day practice. This is followed by a detailed introduction to the practical skill of taking and interpreting a family history. Genetic theory is introduced, with chapters covering subjects such as basic biology and laboratory techniques currently available. These may help set the clinical scenarios in context but are not essential to understanding subsequent chapters. Risk assessment, including types of test available, is described, followed by the various modes of inheritance together with the possibilities and options for families, illustrated throughout with the use of case studies. Specific issues of ethnicity and ethical issues are also addressed. The development of genetic counselling as a profession for healthcare professionals and future developments in the field of clinical genetics are explored and the final chapter focuses on integrating genetics into patient care pathways.

A glossary is included to explain common terms in use throughout the book. It is also useful as a quick reference guide. Finally, a list of relevant web sites is also provided.

The book can be read as a whole but healthcare professionals may wish to dip into individual chapters to address a specific query.

Clinical application of genetic knowledge is coming to be of increasing importance in every area of life and healthcare professionals are therefore more frequently being asked to provide information. This book aims to help the professional feel more confident in dealing with queries and to allow them to know where to go for further advice.

1 The Scientific and Clinical Discoveries That are Used to Provide Current Patient Care

PETER FARNDON

Patients and families today can take advantage of much scientific and clinical knowledge about the mechanisms which cause human disorders, including the differing contributions made by our genes and the environment. Understanding genetic factors can explain patterns of affected people in a family and make predictions about the likelihood of others developing a condition. For some disorders, information about a person's genetic constitution can be used to inform the most appropriate therapy.

Our ability to use genetic knowledge and technology in modern medical care is the result of discoveries made over the last hundred years or so. It was in 1905 that William Bateson first coined the word 'genetics' to include the study of heredity and variation. There have been slow steady advances built on painstaking work, but also giant leaps, particularly relating to advances in the technology of handling and interrogating DNA.

Rather than present a history of genetics as a timeline starting from the earliest discoveries to the present, this chapter will start with a clinical scenario and trace back the discoveries which had to be made in order to enable the study of heredity and variation to enhance clinical care.

A FAMILY WITH BREAST CANCER

The diagram shows in pictorial form a family where several women have had breast cancer.

Breast cancer is a very common condition: one in nine British women develop it. That several women are affected in the pattern shown could be due to a chance clustering but this would be unusual so the family pattern warrants further consideration. Breast cancer is a disease which on the whole affects older women; the

Genetics in Practice: A clinical approach for healthcare practitioners Edited by Jo Haydon
© 2007 John Wiley & Sons, Ltd

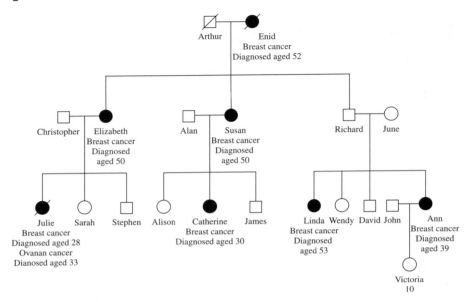

Pedigree 1.1

women in this family were at a much younger age than might be expected from the population incidence.

Ann decided that she would consult her family doctor to determine whether there might be an increased probability of her daughter developing breast cancer. The family doctor was also concerned about the early onset and numbers of women affected and so he referred her to a clinical genetics department. After considerable discussion, Ann undertook a DNA test. This showed a change in the DNA code of one of the two copies of the BRCA1 gene, which resulted in that copy of the gene not working correctly. As a change in the gene associated with a predisposition to breast cancer had been found, other members of the family were offered testing for the same change, and surveillance as appropriate. The genetics department knew that the change in the gene occurred in an area which was also associated with an increased risk for ovarian cancer, and so women in the family were also recommended to undergo regular screening for early detection and treatment for ovarian cancer.

Many families, like Ann's, are now able to obtain genetic information which directly affects management. But what have we had to learn about genetics to be able to offer this service?

These are some of the questions that we need to answer:

- How can we record details of family history in pictorial form?
- Are there particular patterns of affected people which suggest that a condition might be inherited?

- How can we determine the risks to other members of a family?
- How can we explain the particular patterns of people affected with genetic disorders?
- How do we know that DNA is the chemical which carries hereditary instructions/genetic information?
- How can we handle and copy DNA in the laboratory?
- How was the gene responsible found?
- How can we identify changes in a gene, and how do we know that these are responsible for a condition?
- How is DNA transferred from generation to generation?
- How are genetics services provided for patients?

HOW CAN WE RECORD DETAILS OF FAMILY HISTORY IN PICTORIAL FORM?

Although family history information can be recorded in many ways, the genetic relationships between individuals in a family are often best appreciated by drawing a family pedigree.

The term pedigree comes from the French *pied du gru* ('crane's foot'), because the lines descending from parents to children resemble the spindly foot of a crane. During the 1900s, several different forms of symbols were in use, such as depicting everyone in a pedigree by a circle, and then placing arrows pointing upwards (for a male) and downwards (for a female). Genealogical (rather than medical) pedigrees were often drawn as a tree. The current symbols (squares for males, circles for females, blocked in if a person is affected) have the advantages of being clear and preventing ambiguity. They are accepted internationally (see Chapter 2).

DO PARTICULAR PATTERNS OF AFFECTED PEOPLE SUGGEST THAT A CONDITION MIGHT BE INHERITED?

Over the centuries families, scientists and physicians have recognised that certain characteristics cluster in families. In biblical times, Jewish law recognised that if there was a family history of two previous brothers or two maternal cousins dying from bleeding after circumcision, a boy could not be circumcised. The familial pattern of haemophilia was noted in a newspaper account in the 1790s.

Pierre de Maupertuis showed from pedigree studies that polydactyly (extra digits on hands and/or feet) and albinism were inherited in different ways. In 1814, a British doctor, Joseph Adams, also recognised different mechanisms of inheritance in his 'Treatise on the supposed hereditary properties of diseases'. Pliny Earle, a psychiatrist in Philadelphia, delineated the inheritance pattern of colour blindness on the basis of his own family in 1845.

Although particular pedigree patterns were being described for certain traits and diseases, it was not until the early 1900s that an understanding of the physical basis responsible for them became possible. This required the recognition of the movement of chromosomes in cell division, together with the laws of inheritance as discovered by Mendel.

EXPLAINING PATTERNS OF INHERITANCE: THE CONTRIBUTION OF MENDEL

In humans, one has to observe naturally occurring unions, which give relatively small numbers of offspring. Gregor Mendel, an Augustinian monk, however, made enormous contributions to our understanding of the segregation of characteristics in offspring through his experiments with plants in the monastery garden.

Mendel (1822–84) was able to look at large numbers of plants and to construct breeding experiments for nine years. He was especially interested in seven easily distinguishable physical characteristics in peas, each of which had two obviously different expressions (for instance round or wrinkled ripe seeds, yellow or green peas, tall or short plants). He noted that some of these physical characteristics, when present in both parents (e.g. short plants), 'bred true' in the offspring. In contrast, some (e.g. tall plants) were not always true-breeding. Some tall plants, when crossed with a short plant or another tall plant, produced only tall plants in the next generation. This suggested that tallness always masked shortness – Mendel thus called the property for tallness 'dominant'. But when certain other tall plants were crossed with each other, about one quarter of the plants in the next generation were short. He called the property for shortness 'recessive'. Mendel suggested that the elementen (or characters) were being passed from one generation to the next in the gametes. Mendel reasoned that the patterns he saw in his breeding experiments could be explained if an individual gamete contained one or other of the parental elementen for the physical characteristic and this was joined with an elementen from the other partner at fertilisation.

Figure 1.1 shows one of Mendel's plant breeding experiments and how the plant's appearance (phenotype) can be explained by the characters it has inherited from its parents (genotype). When a plant has two copies of an identical form of a character, this is called homozygous; when it has different forms of the character, this is called heterozygous.

In 1865, Mendel presented his results to a National History Society (in what is now Brno in the Czech Republic) and his results were published in the society's journal the following year.

Because the physical basis of meiosis had not yet been described, Mendelism had no plausible basis to qualify it over the other possible mechanisms of inheritance being discussed at the time. One, favoured by Mendel's contemporaries, was the idea that characters in offspring blended together.

1 Certain physical characteristics when present in both parents (e.g. short plants) 'breed true' in the offspring.

A cross between two pure-bred short plants – both have two copies of the gene (t) for shortness (they are homozygous)

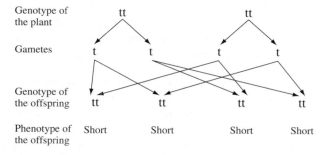

2 Some tall plants, when crossed with a short plant, produce only tall plants in the next generation. This suggested that tallness always masks shortness – a property which Mendel called 'dominant'.

A cross between pure-bred tall and a pure-bred short plant

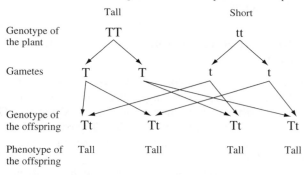

3 When certain tall plants were crossed with each other, about one quarter of the plants in the next generation were short. Mendel called the property for shortness 'recessive'.

A cross between two tall plants, each of which had a gene for tallness (T) and a gene for shortness(t)

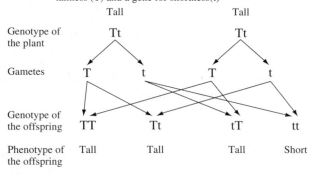

Figure 1.1 Explanations for the Result of Three of Mendel's Experiments

HOW DO WE KNOW IF A DISORDER IS INHERITED IN A MENDELIAN MANNER?

Looking at the Patterns in a Family

The principles which Mendel demonstrated are applicable far beyond his experiments with peas, and to acknowledge his enormous contribution the term 'Mendelian' is applied to patterns of inheritance compatible with the segregation of a pair of characteristics apparently under the control of a single gene.

When Mendel's paper was rediscovered in 1900 it stimulated researchers to repeat and confirm the ratios in other species, and physicians to study inherited diseases, over the years 1900–6. In 1909, the Danish botanist Johannsen renamed Mendel's elementen 'genes' and introduced the terms genotype (genetic constitution) and phenotype (physical characteristics).

Today we use the principles of Mendelism in interpreting pedigree patterns to discover if diseases follow a pattern of dominant or recessive inheritance. We also deduce whether the gene for the disease is likely to be on an autosome or the X chromosome, just as E.B. Wilson predicted in 1911 that colour blindness was a recessive character on an X chromosome because men were affected and related through their unaffected mothers.

Some Conditions are Known to Have a Specific Mode of Inheritance – The Diagnosis Gives the Genetics

William Bateson and Archibald Garrod recognised recessive inheritance of alkaptonuria (a metabolic disorder causing progressive damage to the joints) in 1902, deducing that this was an inherited disorder involving a chemical process. Garrod called this group of diseases 'inborn errors of metabolism'. The pattern of recessive inheritance of alkaptonuria was recognised in 1902; the gene on chromosome 3 responsible was cloned in 1996.

Some people believe that genetic conditions are untreatable, but many metabolic disorders respond well to treatment, particularly dietary measures. For other conditions, enzyme replacement therapy has become available (for instance, in 1991 for type 1 Gaucher disease), although this is usually extremely expensive.

To try to prevent complications by offering early treatment, neonatal screening programmes have been developed. In 1961, Robert Guthrie developed a way to test whether newborn babies have phenylketonuria, a metabolic disorder in which the amino acid phenylalanine builds up in the blood and, if untreated, can cause mental retardation. This was the first neonatal screening programme. Today newborns throughout much of the world are screened for this and other metabolic disorders (such as hypothyroidism) to institute early treatment.

Consulting Databases

To give patients and their families accurate genetic information, it became important to identify and make a catalogue of single genes and their disorders. By 1966, almost 1500 had been identified in a comprehensive catalogue compiled by the famous American physician and geneticist Victor McKusick. This database is now freely available as Online Mendelian Inheritance in Man (OMIM) and in February 2007 contained 17,413 entries.

HOW DOES ONE WORK OUT THE PROBABILITY OF A PERSON BEING AFFECTED OR A CARRIER?

Probabilities of being affected or of being a carrier can be assessed for Mendelian conditions by working out the probability of a person inheriting a particular combination of genes from his or her parents.

Reginald Punnett (1875–1967), a British geneticist, devised a simple aid to take into account all the different combinations of alleles from the mother and the father. The Punnett square is used to predict the probability of possible genotypes occurring in the offspring.

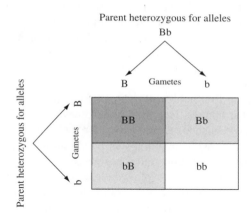

Figure 1.2 Punnett Square

In the example, each parent has the genetic constitution (genotype) Bb. They are thus capable of making gametes that contain either B or b (it is conventional in genetics to use upper case letters to indicate alleles for a dominant character and lower case letters to indicate alleles for a recessive character). The Punnett square shows every possible combination when combining one maternal allele with one paternal allele. In the example, 1/4 of the offspring will have the genetic constitution BB, 1/2 will be Bb and 1/4 will be bb. It is important to note that Punnett squares give only probabilities for genotypes and not phenotypes. The way in which the B and b alleles interact with each to affect the appearance of the offspring depends on how the gene products interact.

HOW ARE GENETIC FACTORS TRANSFERRED FROM GENERATION TO GENERATION?

Although Mendel had identified the patterns of inheritance and suggested the existence of what would become known as the gene, a physical mechanism to explain Mendel's findings had not yet been discovered. The visualisation of chromosomes and the realisation that they could provide a physical basis for what Mendel had described was the next important step.

We now know that the DNA in a single human nucleus would stretch for about 2 m if pulled out in a straight line. To manage and transfer this amount of DNA from cell to cell – and generation to generation – it is organised into chromosomes.

Walther Flemming published a drawing of chromosomes visible in human tumour cells in mitotic cell division in 1882. He described how chromosomes move during the various stages of cell division in salamander embryos. Waldeyer coined the term chromosome in 1888 because of the affinity of the threadlike structures for certain stains (*chroma* = colour, *soma* = body).

In 1902, Theodor Boveri, a German biologist studying sea urchins, and Walter Sutton, an American medical student studying grasshopper cells, proposed independently that chromosomes carried the hereditary factors. Both had observed that during the process of meiotic cell division, each egg or sperm cell produced had only one copy of each chromosome rather than the usual two. The chromosomes segregated into the gametes at meiosis, which explained the segregation of Mendel's factors from generation to generation.

Although Flemming first published a drawing of human chromosomes in 1882, it was considered that humans had 48 chromosomes until 1956, when the correct number of 46 was established, three years after the structure of DNA had been proposed. Experimenting with conditions during chromosome preparation achieved a better spreading and visualisation of the chromosomes. Very soon human disorders were shown to be due to gain or loss of a whole chromosome. Down syndrome was the first in 1959 due to the presence of an additional number 21 chromosome. Other chromosomal syndromes quickly followed, and were named after their investigators: Patau (trisomy 13), Edwards (trisomy 18), Turner (monosomy X) and Klinefelter (47, XXY).

With the understanding of the inheritance of single gene disorders, and the visual proof that some conditions were caused by chromosomal anomalies, some families asked whether it was possible to detect these conditions before birth. It is necessary to obtain genetic material from the foetus and over the years sampling techniques such as amniocentesis and chorionic villus biopsy have been developed (see also Chapter 5).

Initially the chromosomes were stained uniformly but by the early 1970s, special staining techniques had been developed to identify a detailed pattern of dark and light bands on each chromosome. The methods of chromosome preparation were refined, particularly to elongate the chromosomes so that more detailed analysis could be performed. It came to be appreciated that some people have syndromic features and developmental delay associated with small pieces of chromosome being deleted or duplicated. Such microscopic analyses were at the limit of optical resolution and many people felt that cytogenetic analysis would not be able to develop further.

However, by the late 1980s/early 1990s it became possible to label the strands of a specific piece of human DNA with fluorescent dyes and this could be used to show whether the DNA was present and in the correct position in a particular patient. This is called fluorescence in situ hybridisation (FISH) and is described in more detail in Chapter 4. This technique has been so refined that it is now possible to detect small changes in the structure of a chromosome, including the presence or absence of just one gene.

A further development is comparative genomic hybridisation, where probes covering the whole of the genome are used to look for submicroscopic structural variations – duplications and deletions – across all the chromosomes at once. It may be that this will replace microscopic analysis of chromosomes in patients where there is a strong clinical indication that a subtle chromosome anomaly may be present. This technique can also be used to see the pattern of genes active in a particular cancer, which can be used to target therapy.

HOW DO WE KNOW THAT DNA IS THE CHEMICAL WHICH CARRIES HEREDITARY INSTRUCTIONS/GENETIC INFORMATION?

Mendel had identified the patterns of inheritance but the chemical nature of his elementen was not known. Although DNA had been isolated from white cells in pus in bandages and called nuclein (because it came from the nucleus) by Friedrich Miescher in 1867, for some time proteins were considered to be the most likely material to carry the genetic instructions. As DNA was believed to be a simple molecule – of phosphate and nitrogen – how could it carry the complex information required for heredity?

Experiments were conducted in mice in the 1930s in which types of bacteria responsible for pneumonia were subjected to treatments which inactivated either protein or DNA. These experiments showed that in fact it was through the DNA that the mice became infected. This was further confirmed in 1953 (the same year that the structure of DNA was proposed) by Alfred Hershey and Martha Chase, who showed that DNA (and not protein) from a virus could direct a cell to produce multiple copies of the virus.

Two lines of experimental evidence came together in the early 1950s to inspire Watson and Crick to propose the double helix structure of DNA. Erwin Chargaff showed in 1950 that in DNA there are equal amounts of adenine and thymine, and equal amounts of guanine and cytosine, and the proportions are specific to individual species. Rosalind Franklin and Maurice Wilkins at King's College in London had produced X-ray photographs which revealed that DNA had a regularly repeating structure. James Watson and Francis Crick made a three dimensional model which satisfied these findings, and ended their *Nature* paper with the words 'It has not escaped our notice that the specific pairing we have postulated immediately suggests a possible copying mechanism for the genetic material.'

HOW CAN ONLY FOUR LETTERS MAKE A HUMAN?

So now the structure and composition of DNA was known, but how could a chemical containing only four different 'letters' (bases) – A T C G – code for the twenty different amino acids which make up proteins? If an amino acid was coded by a run of three letters, this would give 64 different possible combinations – more than enough to code for the 20 amino acids (see Chapter 3). The project to work out this three letter code gathered pace in the 1960s, so that the complete genetic code was solved by 1966.

Clinically, we need to read the DNA sequence to work out the structure of a protein – for instance whether it is an enzyme or a receptor or a structural protein – in order to help predict the effects that a particular alteration (mutation) may have on a protein, and the effects that this may produce in a disease.

HOW DOES DNA COPY ITSELF TO PASS ITSELF ON?

A remarkable feature of DNA is that one strand acts as a template for its partner strand. Pulling the double-stranded DNA apart yields two single strands of DNA. By filling in the missing strand of each, following the Watson–Crick binding rules (A to T, T to A, G to C, C to G), the original double-stranded DNA has made two exact copies. In the laboratory, we can therefore make many copies of a particular sequence of DNA in which we are interested. Knowing a DNA sequence means that the complementary sequence can be predicted and used to make a DNA 'probe', such as those used for FISH.

Although copying DNA usually makes exact copies, occasionally errors occur, resulting in alterations (mutations) to the sequence, which cause genetic diseases.

WHY DO WE NEED TO HANDLE AND COPY DNA IN THE LABORATORY?

To analyse human DNA, it usually has to be cut into smaller pieces, and multiple copies must be made of the particular DNA pieces which are to undergo laboratory analysis. Both these steps have required specific technology to be developed.

A breakthrough came when a group of enzymes was discovered in 1962 which would cut DNA into a pattern of pieces specific to each person. This laid the path to using such DNA patterns as markers to identify genes responsible for diseases (such as Huntington disease, cystic fibrosis and Duchenne muscular dystrophy) and for diagnosis by following the inheritance of a particular piece of DNA through a family.

Originally, recombinant DNA technology was used to synthesise multiple copies of a particular piece of DNA in bacteria or viruses, but this was a very time-consuming and tedious process. The next breakthrough occurred in 1985 when the polymerase chain reaction was invented to produce multiple copies of a specific short segment of DNA, for which Mullis received the Nobel prize (see Chapter 4).

HOW IS THE LOCATION OF A GENE FOUND?

Let us consider the example of how the gene responsible for the predisposition to breast cancer was found.

Breast cancer is common – a British woman has a lifetime risk of 1 in 9 – so when several relatives have breast cancer this may be due to chance. However, there appear to be some families where many more women are affected than would be predicted by chance, and where the women are affected at an earlier age than is usual. Such families suggest the possibility that there is an inherited cause for the susceptibility to breast cancer.

To try to identify possible breast-cancer susceptibility genes, the patterns of affected people in 1500 families were reviewed, and statistical analysis suggested that 4–5% of breast cancer was associated with inherited factors. Of the 1500 families, 23 where the condition appeared to be inherited as an autosomal dominant condition took part in a study to determine whether it was being inherited with any particular chromosome marker. The study suggested that there might be a breast-cancer gene on the long arm of chromosome 17, which was called BRCA1. An international collaborative study was then set up with a new set of 214 families and the results were confirmed. This study narrowed down the area on chromosome 17 in which the gene was likely to be found – DNA from the area was extracted, copied and sequenced to find candidate genes. The sequence of BRCA1 was identified in 1994; it was confirmed as a gene for breast cancer susceptibility because mutations compatible with disrupting the action of the gene were found in women from families with this type of inherited breast cancer. Other genes have also been implicated using similar 'gene tracking' methods.

Such a study involves recognising a familial pattern, determining how the condition might be inherited, copying and examining DNA, and determining that mutations found in a candidate gene are compatible with altering gene function.

For other conditions where the inheritance is known, a linkage study can be undertaken using families with the appropriate structure of affected people. For instance, the first genetic disease to be mapped to a chromosome (chromosome 4) using DNA polymorphisms was Huntington disease in 1983. Using the cloning techniques available then, it took 10 years before the gene was isolated in 1993, the result of a collaboration of 58 researchers in 6 research groups.

Other gene discoveries are shown in Table 1.1.

Table 1.1 Gene Discoveries in Common Genetic Conditions

Disorder	Chromosome	Year gene isolated and genetic code read
Duchenne muscular dystrophy	X	1986
Cystic fibrosis	7	1989
Myotonic dystrophy	19	1992
Huntington disease	4	1993
Breast cancer, familial, type 1	17	1994
Breast cancer, familial, type 2	13	1995

HOW CAN WE IDENTIFY CHANGES IN A GENE?

Although current practice interrogates DNA for changes in genetic diseases, the first reported specific cause of a genetic disorder came in 1956, when experiments using protein chemistry showed that the sickle cell beta globin has a substitution of one amino acid for another (glutamic acid replaced by valine) at amino acid position number six in the protein.

A gene may be suspected of being the one responsible for a particular genetic condition because:

- It has been isolated following information from a linkage study.
- A homologue (similar gene) in another organism has been associated with the same disease.
- A search has been made for genes which have particular characteristics that are predicted to cause a disease.

The proof that a gene is the one causing a particular disorder is that alterations are found in the structure or DNA code of the gene (mutations) which result in disordered function. Therefore, we usually need to be able to read the DNA sequence of the gene in someone with the disorder and compare it with the gene in people without the disorder.

READING THE DNA SEQUENCE

The most commonly used DNA sequencing technique was developed by Fred Sanger in 1977. The technique, which reads the letters sequentially, is the one normally used for DNA sequencing in hospital genetics laboratories. In 2007, there are some exciting new advances which offer the promise of sequencing very long stretches of DNA very quickly using single molecule sequencing. The long-term aim of the US National Human Genome Research Institute is to achieve technology which will sequence an individual person's entire genome for $1000.

HOW DO WE KNOW THAT CHANGES IN A GENE ARE RESPONSIBLE FOR A GENETIC CONDITION?

When DNA sequencing has provided the printout of the base sequence of the DNA segments being investigated, this is compared, letter by letter, with the usual gene sequence to spot any differences. Then an opinion has to be formed as to whether any change in the sequence is likely to cause a severe problem in the activity or function of the gene product (see Chapter 3).

HOW ARE GENETICS INFORMATION AND SERVICES PROVIDED FOR PATIENTS?

The first UK genetic clinic was set up at the Hospital for Sick Children, Great Ormond Street in 1946 by Dr J. Fraser Roberts, who was joined by Dr Cedric Carter in 1952 as part-time research fellow in genetics. Dr Carter became a member of the scientific staff of the Medical Research Council's Genetic Unit when this was established in the Institute of Child Health in 1957. He was appointed consultant geneticist at the Hospital for Sick Children in 1958 and at Queen Charlotte's Hospital in 1973.

The term 'genetic counselling' was coined by Sheldon Reed, who was one of the medical geneticists who started their careers as biologists. He turned to human genetics in 1947, when he became director of the Dight Institute for Human Genetics at the University of Minnesota. Immediately he began to receive questions from physicians about genetic problems they had encountered. As a wide range of questions continued, he kept looking for a term that would describe what he was doing. He presented the concept of 'genetic counselling' at the First International Congress of Human Genetics, in Copenhagen, in 1956.

Originally, most genetic counselling and research was undertaken in university departments, often by enthusiastic physicians and scientists from other specialties. In the 1980s, genetic medicine became a recognised specialty in the NHS, with recognised specialist training to become a consultant clinical geneticist. Regional genetic centres developed, encompassing academic activities and research and providing a clinical and laboratory service serving populations of 2–6 million. Clinical and laboratory services worked closely together and developed 'hub and spoke' systems with clinics in district hospitals. They provide access to the latest developments, clinical diagnosis, laboratory (DNA and chromosomal) diagnosis, genetic counselling and genetic management of extended families. In the 1990s, the work of the regional centres expanded greatly, particularly in working with colleagues in primary care and other specialities to determine which families with breast/ovarian and colon cancer were most likely to have a Mendelian form of predisposition to cancer, and offering genetic testing, surveillance and management.

POINTS FOR REFLECTION

- The reason we are able to provide the services available to patients is a direct result of teamwork between scientists and clinical services.
- In genetics it is important to recognise that when the genetic basis for an individual patient's disorder is understood, it can give important new insights into the biology of mankind.
- Do you know how to obtain specialist genetic advice applicable to your patients?

2 The Family History

JO HAYDON

Genetic counselling is a process comprising several components aimed at enabling the individual or family to:

1. comprehend the medical facts, including the diagnosis, probable course of the disorder, and the available management
2. appreciate the way heredity contributes to the disorder, and the risk of recurrence in specified relatives
3. understand the alternatives for dealing with the risk of recurrence
4. choose the course of action which seems to them appropriate in view of their risk, their family goals and their ethical and religious standards, and to act in accordance with that decision
5. make the best possible adjustment to the disorder in an affected family member and/or the risk of recurrence of that disorder (Ad Hoc Committee on Genetic Counseling, 1975).

An accurate diagnosis is therefore essential and although there may be a laboratory test available to assist in this, the single most important tool is the record of the family history (also referred to as a pedigree). The pattern of affected individuals within a family may provide an important clue as to the diagnosis, the probable inheritance pattern and the risks for family members. This in turn may reduce delay in diagnosis and possibly eliminate the need for unpleasant, expensive and time-consuming investigations for those family members not at risk. The ability to take an accurate family history is essential for professionals working in the field of clinical genetics. It is also increasingly important for other health professionals as the demand from their clients for genetic information increases. Recording an accurate family history can avoid unnecessary referral to the clinical genetics services, therefore reducing client anxiety for those not at risk and reducing delay for those for whom referral would be appropriate.

Obtaining this information is not only important for accurate diagnosis; it also helps to develop a rapport with the client, which enables the client to feel confident in revealing what may be sensitive information. In presenting the information, the

Genetics in Practice: A clinical approach for healthcare practitioners   Edited by Jo Haydon
© 2007 John Wiley & Sons, Ltd

client may also provide useful information about family dynamics and relationships with individuals within the family. The family's perceptions of the disease and its inheritance and specific concerns may also be clarified.

All the relevant information may not be available immediately and further details about the family may need to be obtained by the client before the family tree can be accurately drawn. Examining the pedigree with the family may be helpful in explaining the method of inheritance and in clarifying those individuals who may be at risk of becoming affected or of being carriers.

GUIDELINES FOR TAKING A FAMILY HISTORY AND DRAWING A PEDIGREE

1. It is helpful to follow a pattern each time a family history is taken to ensure that all the relevant information is obtained. In this way it is less likely that important details will be omitted.
2. Standard pedigree symbols are used to enable others to interpret the information correctly (see Table 2.1).
3. For each individual on the pedigree, record the full name (including the maiden name of women where appropriate) and the date of birth. If the full date of birth is not known, record the year of birth rather than the age as it may be necessary to refer back to the pedigree at some time in the future. Details of health problems should be noted, including the age at diagnosis where appropriate. It may be useful to ask, 'Has *x* ever needed treatment in hospital?' to avoid previous episodes of ill health being omitted.
4. Start in the middle of the sheet with the client, then add their partner (the usual convention is to place the male partner on the left) and their children (in birth order with the firstborn on the left).
5. Ask if the client or their partner have children from previous relationships and add these to the pedigree.
6. Remember to ask about children who have died, also stillbirths and miscarriages (this applies to all adults in the pedigree). You might do this by asking, 'Did you lose any babies or have any other pregnancies?' Information about the length of gestation (i.e. number of weeks of pregnancy) for pregnancy losses should be recorded. If an individual is currently pregnant, the LMP (date of last menstrual period) and/or EDD (expected date of delivery) should be recorded.
7. Information should then be obtained about the client's siblings, nieces and nephews, parents, aunts and uncles. It is important to include family members who have died, recording the date (or year) and cause of death when known.
8. Similar information should then be obtained about the client's partner's family.
9. Affected individuals are represented by shading in their symbol. If there are several diagnoses in the family, different shadings will be required and a key should be provided to explain these.

Table 2.1 Pedigree Symbols

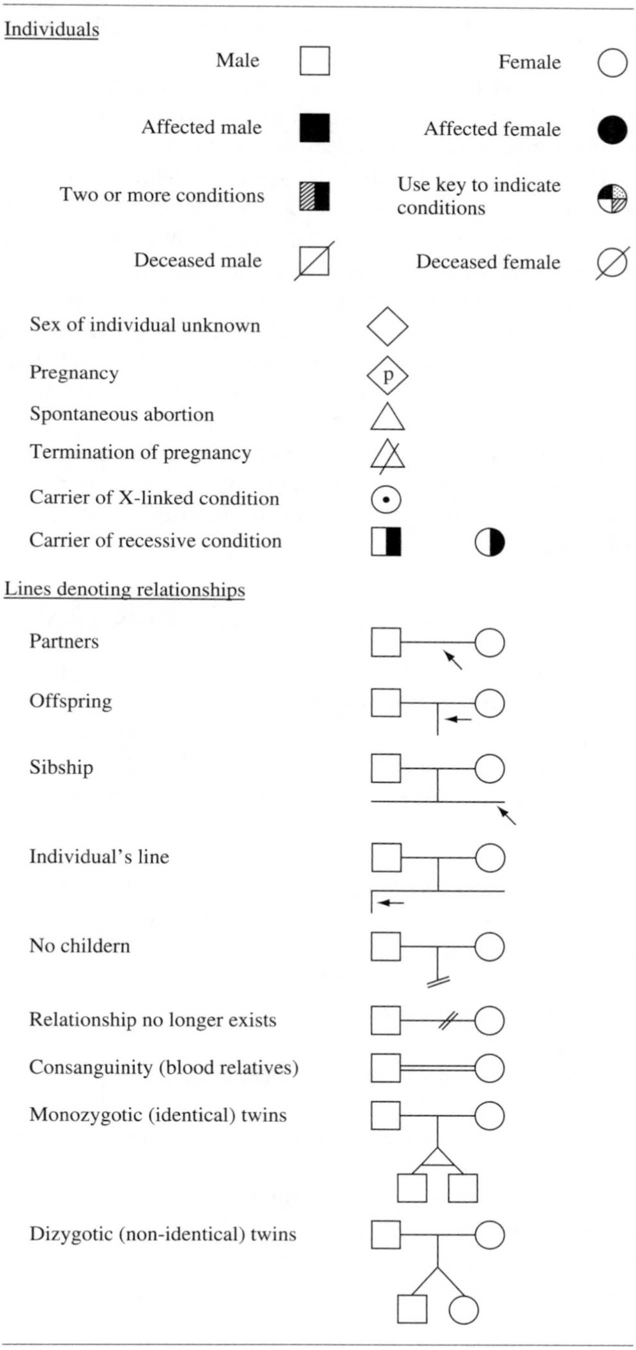

Individuals

Male	☐	Female	○
Affected male	■	Affected female	●
Two or more conditions	▨	Use key to indicate conditions	◉
Deceased male	⧄	Deceased female	⦰

Sex of individual unknown ◇

Pregnancy ⟨p⟩

Spontaneous abortion △

Termination of pregnancy △̸

Carrier of X-linked condition ⊙

Carrier of recessive condition ◧ ◐

Lines denoting relationships

Partners

Offspring

Sibship

Individual's line

No childern

Relationship no longer exists

Consanguinity (blood relatives)

Monozygotic (identical) twins

Dizygotic (non-identical) twins

10. Ask about consanguinity within the family, as this may be relevant for autosomal recessive disorders. This should be done sensitively; you might ask, 'Were you related before marriage?' or 'Do you share any common surnames in the family?'

11. Record details about both sides of the family, even if the disorder appears to be obviously affecting one side. There may be another genetic condition that could easily be missed if a full history is not obtained. It is also important that the partner on whose side the disorder seems to segregate is not made to feel guilty or to think that anyone is apportioning blame.

12. When you think you have completed the family history, ask the client if they have any further information to give you that they think might be relevant.

13. Numbering the individuals may be helpful in a large family where several people share a common first name as well as their surname. If such numbering is necessary, start at the top of the pedigree and number each generation using Roman numerals. Number the individuals in each generation, starting on the left hand side, using ordinal numbers.

14. When the pedigree is complete, the individual recording the information should record their name and the date on which the information was obtained. The name of the person/people from whom the information was obtained should also be recorded.

A PRACTICAL EXAMPLE OF TAKING A FAMILY HISTORY

Jenny and Phillip have been referred for genetic counselling several months after the death of their son, Robert (DOB 05/02/2007), aged two months. The genetic counsellor has spent some time discussing the events leading up to Robert's death and the bereavement issues that the couple is currently experiencing. At an appropriate point the counsellor moves on to taking the family history in the following manner:

Counsellor: 'Are you now ready for me to take some details about your families?'
Jenny: 'Yes, yes that's fine.' (Phillip nods in agreement.)
C: 'Jenny, what is your date of birth?'
Jenny: 'It's the 3rd December, 1976.'
C: 'What was your maiden name?'
Jenny: 'Roberts.'
C: 'Have you had any major illnesses or operations?'
Jenny: 'No.'
C: 'You've told me about Robert and how devastated you have been since his death. Have you got any other children?'
Jenny: 'Yes, we've got Emma, our daughter.'
C: 'What is Emma's date of birth?'
Jenny: 'She was born in 2003, on the 16th March.'
C: 'Do you have any worries about her health or development?'

Jenny: 'Oh no. She's always been very healthy and she's a bright little girl.'

C: 'Good. Have you had any other pregnancies apart from Emma and Robert?'

Jenny: 'Yes. I had two miscarriages, between Emma and Robert, one in November 2004, and the other was in June 2005.'

C: 'Do you remember how far the pregnancies had progressed when this happened?'

Jenny: 'Yes, it was about 10 weeks with the first and 9 weeks with the second one.'

C: 'You must have been very anxious when you became pregnant the fourth time.'

Jenny: 'Yes, we didn't relax until I had my scan at 19 weeks, then we thought everything would be all right.'

C: 'So when Robert was born and he had some obvious problems it must have come as quite a shock to you.'

Jenny: 'Yes, it was terrible.'

(C allows several moments of quiet reflection before continuing.)

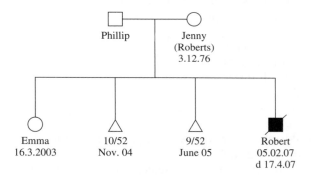

Pedigree 2.1

C: 'Have you had any children by a previous partner?'

Jenny: 'No.'

C: 'Have you got any brothers or sisters?'

Jenny: 'I've got a brother, Adrian.'

C: 'What's Adrian's date of birth?'

Jenny: '7th September, 1979.'

C: 'Has he ever had any major illnesses or operations?'

Jenny: 'Only his appendix when he was about 10.'

C: 'Has Adrian got a partner?'

Jenny: 'Yes, he's married to Susie.'

C: 'Do you know her date of birth?'

Jenny: 'Yes, it's 19th December, 1980.'

C: 'Have they got any children?'

Jenny: 'No, but Susie has had two miscarriages.'

C: 'Do you know how early in the pregnancy they occurred?'

Jenny: 'I think they were both at about 10–11 weeks, something like that.'

C: 'Do you have any other brothers or sisters?'

Jenny: 'No. I did have a sister, Fleur, but she died soon after birth.'

C: 'Do you know what caused her death?'

Jenny: 'Mum doesn't say much about her but she did say Fleur had lots of problems. I think she said that she wasn't properly formed but I don't like to ask her much because she gets upset.'

C: 'I can understand that. Did your mother have any other pregnancies that you're aware of?'

Jenny: 'Yes, when I had the first miscarriage mum said that her first two pregnancies miscarried.'

C: 'So your mum had five pregnancies altogether?'

Jenny: 'Yes, that's right'

C: 'Are your parents still alive and well?'

Jenny: 'My mother is but my father died four years ago.'

C: 'What is your mother's name?'

Jenny: 'Janet.'

C: 'And her date of birth?'

Jenny: '15th March, 1950.'

C: 'Has she ever had any serious illnesses?'

Jenny: 'No.'

C: 'What was your father's first name?'

Jenny: 'Cyril.'

C: 'You said he died four years ago; do you remember his date of birth and the date on which he died?'

Jenny: 'Yes, his birthday was 20th September and he was born in 1946. He died on 31st October, 2003.'

C: 'What caused his death?'

Jenny: 'He had a heart attack.'

C: 'Did your parents have many brothers and sisters?'

Jenny: 'No, they were both only children.'

C: 'Phillip, I would like to ask you some details about yourself and your family. First of all, what is your date of birth?'

Phillip: '5th June, 1975.'

C: 'And have you ever had any serious illnesses or operations?'

Philip: 'No.'

C: 'Have you had any children by a previous partner?'

Phillip: 'Yes. I've got twin boys by my first wife.'

C: 'What are the boys' names?'

Phillip: 'Jordan and Ben.'

C: 'And their date of birth?'

Phillip: '26th September, 1999'

C: 'Are they identical twins, do you know?'

Phillip: 'No, no they're not.'

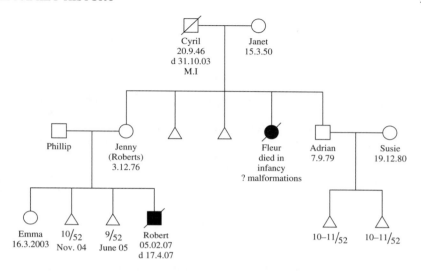

Pedigree 2.2

C: 'Have they had any problems with their health?'

Phillip: 'No. They're both healthy and they seem to be doing very well at school so we've had no worries about them.'

C: 'Have you got any brothers or sisters?'

Phillip: 'No, I'm an only child.'

C: 'Are your parents both alive?'

Phillip: 'Yes, they are.'

C: 'What's your father's name and date of birth?'

Phillip: He's George and his birthday is 12th April, 1950.'

C: 'Has he ever had any serious illnesses or operations?'

Phillip: 'No. He's always been very fit.'

C: 'Does he have any brothers or sisters?'

Phillip: 'Not as far as he knows. He was adopted and he doesn't know anything about his family.'

C: 'What's your mother's name and date of birth?'

Phillip: 'She's called Emily and her birthday is on 13th August, 1954.'

C: Has she had any serious illnesses or operations?

Phillip: 'She had a heart attack two years ago but she's been very well since then.'

C: 'Does she have any brothers or sisters?'

Phillip: 'I think she had but we don't have any contact with them. My mum fell out with them years ago. When she got married, I think.'

Now that a full pedigree has been obtained, we can look at the features that are most obvious to us. There are two children who have had severe, and possibly

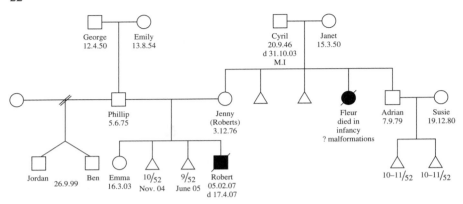

Pedigree 2.3

similar, abnormalities. There are also three women who have had several miscarriages each and, although we know that miscarriage is common, within a family this is a higher incidence than might be expected. By looking at this pedigree, the genetics team will suspect a possible reason for these problems within the family and order the most appropriate test to confirm their suspicions (we will return to Jenny and Phillip later in the chapter.) We can therefore see why it is important to be able to interpret pedigree findings.

INTERPRETATION OF INFORMATION

Having drawn the family tree, it may be possible to determine whether the disease is likely to be genetic by looking at the pattern that emerges. Modes of inheritance have significant characteristics that result in different patterns.

AUTOSOMAL DOMINANT INHERITANCE (SEE CHAPTER 7)

If a condition is inherited in an autosomal dominant fashion, one copy of the gene is normal and the second copy is altered. An individual only has to inherit one altered copy to be affected. Therefore, offspring of an affected individual have a 1 in 2 (50%) risk of having inherited the altered gene. Examples of some dominant disorders include adult polycystic kidney disease, Huntington disease, neurofibromatosis and familial adenomatous polyposis.

Typical Features of an Autosomal Dominant Pedigree

- Usually involves more than one generation.
- Males and females affected in roughly equal numbers.

- All forms of transmission observed (i.e. male to male, female to female, male to female and female to male).
- An affected individual may have unaffected offspring.

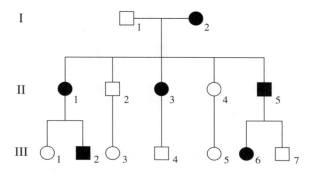

Figure 2.1 A Typical Autosomal Dominant Pedigree. If the disorder in this family manifests itself by adulthood, and all the individuals in generations I and II have reached that stage, which individuals in generation III are still at risk of becoming affected? (*Answers: III.1, 4 & 7.*)

AUTOSOMAL RECESSIVE INHERITANCE (SEE CHAPTER 8)

If a condition is inherited in an autosomal recessive fashion, both copies of the gene must be altered for the individual to be affected. A person affected with an autosomal recessive disorder has inherited one altered copy of the gene from each parent. It is the absence of a normal copy that causes them to be affected. The parents will have one normal copy of the gene and one altered copy of the gene. They are known as gene carriers and are usually healthy, as one normal copy of the gene is sufficient for adequate cell function.

Each child of two carrier parents has a 25% risk of being affected, a 50% risk of being healthy but a carrier and a 25% risk of being healthy and not a carrier. Examples of some autosomal recessive disorders include cystic fibrosis, sickle cell disorders, thalassemia and phenylketonuria.

Typical Features of an Autosomal Recessive Disorder

- Usually affects individuals in a single sibship (i.e. brothers and sisters) in one generation.
- Neither parent affected.
- Males and females affected.
- There may be consanguinity in the parents (i.e. partners who are also blood relatives).

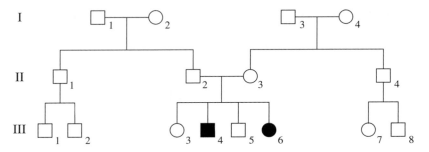

Figure 2.2 A Typical Autosomal Recessive Pedigree. Which individuals in this pedigree *must* be carriers (referred to as obligate carriers) and which individuals *might* be carriers? (*Answers: obligate carriers: II.2 & 3; possible carriers: I.1, 2, 3 & 4; II.1 & 4; III.3 & 5.*)

X-LINKED INHERITANCE (SEE CHAPTER 9)

If a condition is inherited in an x-linked fashion, the altered gene is carried on the X chromosome.

In an X-linked *recessive* condition only one normal copy of the gene is required for adequate cell function. Females have two X chromosomes and therefore have two copies of the gene. Men have one X chromosome and therefore only have one copy of the gene. If a male carries the altered gene on his X chromosome he does not have a normal copy of the gene and is therefore affected with the condition. All his sons will be normal as they inherit his Y chromosome and their X chromosome comes from their mother. All his daughters will be obligate carriers. A female who has one altered copy of the gene also has a normal copy on her other X chromosome and is therefore a carrier but not usually affected (a female with only one X chromosome (Turner syndrome, see Chapter 6) or with skewed inactivation of her X chromosomes (see Chapter 9) may have a milder form of the disorder). Each of her daughters has a 1 in 2 (50%) risk of being a carrier and each of her sons has a 1 in 2 (50%) risk of being affected. The overall risk to her offspring is therefore 1 in 4 (25%). Examples of some X-linked recessive disorders include Duchenne muscular dystrophy, Fragile X syndrome and haemophilia.

Typical Features of an X-Linked Recessive Pedigree

- Usually more than one generation affected.
- Males affected almost exclusively.
- Transmitted through carrier females to their sons.
- Affected males are linked through unaffected female (i.e. female's brother and son affected).
- No male to male transmission.
- Daughters of affected males are always carriers.

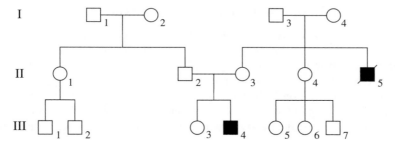

Figure 2.3 A Typical X-Linked Recessive Pedigree. Which females in this pedigree are *obligate* carriers and which females *may* be carriers? (*Answers: obligate carriers: I.4 & II.3; possible carriers: II.4 & III.3.*)

In an X-linked *dominant* disorder an individual only has to inherit one altered copy of the gene to be affected. Only a few disorders are known to be inherited in an X-linked dominant manner. In these disorders (e.g. vitamin D resistant rickets), males are more severely affected than females (who also have one normal copy of the gene). In some X-linked dominant conditions the affected males are so severely affected that spontaneous abortion is usual and only affected females are seen (e.g. incontinentia pigmenti).

Typical Features of an X-Linked Dominant Pedigree

- Males and females are affected but affected females occur more frequently than affected males.
- Females are usually less severely affected than males.
- Affected females can transmit the disorder to male and female children, while affected males transmit the disorder only to their daughters, all of whom are affected.

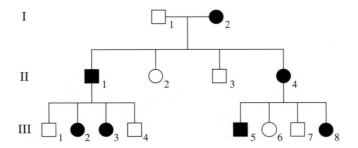

Figure 2.4 A Typical X-Linked Dominant Pedigree.

CHROMOSOMAL ABNORMALITIES (SEE CHAPTER 6)

Now let us return to Jenny and Phillip's family tree (see Pedigree 2.3).

The main features in this pedigree are: recurrent miscarriages in several family members and several children born with abnormalities. They do not fit the pattern of any of the single gene disorders previously described.

A chromosome test on Robert had shown that he had carried some extra chromosome material, and blood tests on Jenny and Philip showed that Jenny carried a chromosome rearrangement known as a balanced translocation (see Chapter 6).

Typical Features of a Chromosomal Pedigree

- Recurrent miscarriages.
- Unexplained infertility.
- Two or more major birth defects in a child.
- Several children born with abnormalities.
- Unexplained developmental delay.

POTENTIAL PROBLEMS TO BE AWARE OF WHEN RECORDING THE PEDIGREE

MISINFORMATION

When asking an individual about other members of their family or their partner's family, the accuracy of the information obtained will depend on the accuracy of the individual's recall and the information known within the family. When taking a pedigree from individuals from different branches of the same family it is not unusual to find some discrepancy in the information obtained.

When accuracy of diagnosis in a reported affected relative will affect the advice to be given to the client, it is important to request permission to contact the relevant family member for permission to obtain their medical records. This can be particularly important in families where there is reputed to be a family history of cancer. It is not uncommon for tumours in the abdominal region (including the uterus and ovaries) to be referred to as 'stomach' cancer.

CONFIDENTIALITY

Individuals from different branches of a family are often seen on separate occasions by the genetic team. It may be that not all the information acquired from one individual is common knowledge amongst other members of that family. One set of case notes is usually kept for the whole family, with a separate section for each individual seen. Care must be taken to ensure that an individual cannot see, from the case notes, which other family members have been in contact with the genetics department. To protect individuals' confidentiality it is wise to take a pedigree from each person seen without showing which other family members are affected, unless that information is given by the consultand (person requiring genetic counselling).

COMPLICATED FAMILY PATTERNS

It is now common to find that an individual has had a number of partners. It is useful to number the partners in order of partnership and to record the surnames of children from each partnership. It is also important to clarify whether sibs share the same parents, are half-sibs (and in these cases, to clearly identify whether the mother or father is the common parent) or are biologically unrelated step-sibs.

When recording adopted children, it is important to differentiate between children adopted into the family (i.e. not biologically related) and those adopted out, about whom no further information may be available.

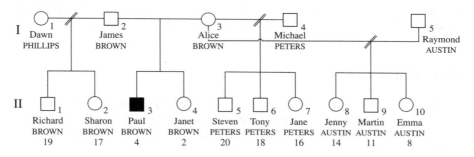

Pedigree 2.4

James and Alice Brown have been referred for genetic counselling because of problems with their son, Paul (II.3).

In this family, Paul and Janet Brown (II.3 & II.4) are *half-siblings* of Richard and Sharon Brown (II.1 & II.2), Steven, Tony and Jane Peters (II.5, II.6, II.7), and Jenny, Martin and Emma Austin (II.8, II.9, & II.10).

Richard and Sharon Brown (II.1 & II.2) are *not biologically related* to their *step-siblings* Steven, Tony and Jane Peters (II.5, II.6, II.7) and Jenny, Martin and Emma Austin (II.8, II.9, & II.10).

If Paul is found to have an autosomal dominant condition, and his father, James Brown, is also found to be affected, who else would be at risk of being affected in this family? (*Answer: II.1, 2 & 4.*)

If Paul is found to have an autosomal recessive condition, who else in the family might be affected and who would be at risk of being carriers? (*Answer: possibly affected: II.4; possible carriers: all second generation i.e. children of James and Alice, James and Dawn, Alice and Michael, Alice and Raymond.*)

If Paul is found to have an X-linked recessive disorder which presents in the first five years of life, who else in the family might be affected? Who might be a carrier for the condition? (*Answer: affected: no one; carrier: I.3; II.4,7,8, & 10.*)

SENSITIVITY OF INFORMATION

It may not be necessary to record sensitive information that has no bearing on the pattern of inheritance. For example, previous terminations of pregnancy not related to the condition being dealt with, or issues regarding paternity not relating to potentially at-risk individuals may not need to be recorded on the pedigree. A record may be kept in the individual's notes without this being entered on the pedigree, which may be seen by other family members.

PHRASING OF QUESTIONS

It is important to ask open-ended questions. Asking, 'Has x ever had any serious illnesses or operations?' or 'Has x ever needed hospital admission?' may elicit a different response than asking, 'Is x well?' On one occasion when taking a pedigree, the author was told that an individual's brother was well but subsequently discovered that he had previously had a kidney removed!

POINTS FOR REFLECTION

- Information obtained from drawing the family tree may be useful in determining the mode of inheritance. Consider the possible pitfalls in interpretation.
- The pictorial representation of the family history in a pedigree format is a useful tool in explaining inheritance to families.
- The pictorial representation is also useful in determining which other family members may be at risk of becoming affected by, or carriers for, a disorder.
- Taking a family history allows the professional an opportunity to gain insight into the family's dynamics and may raise other issues that need to be addressed.
- How easy would it be for you to draw up your own detailed family tree?

REFERENCE

Ad Hoc Committee on Genetic Counseling American Society for Human Genetics (1975) Genetic counselling. *Am J Hum Genet*, **27**, 240–2.

3 Basic Biology

TESSA WEBB AND JO HAYDON

Cells are the basic structural and functional building blocks of all living organisms. A human being is constructed from about 10^{14} living eukaryotic cells. Cells are bounded by a membrane which maintains the integrity of the cell and allows the transport of molecules such as nutrients into and out of it. The cell membrane consists of thin layers of lipids and proteins which allow passage by forming channels. Hereditary material is encoded by DNA, packed into rod-like structures called chromosomes, contained within a nucleus which is bounded by a nuclear membrane and surrounded by cytoplasm. Cytoplasm is a fluid containing the complex molecules necessary for cell survival and a series of organelles (specialised structures contained within a body cell), each performing a specific function or activity for the cell. Mitochondria, which are the power houses of the cell and contain their own DNA, are also found within the cytoplasm.

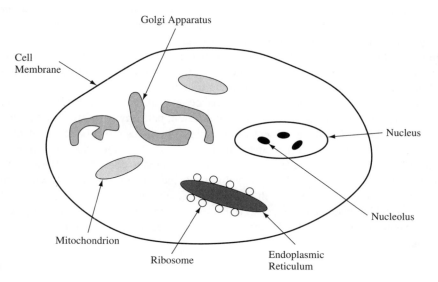

Figure 3.1 Eukaryotic Cell

Genetics in Practice: A clinical approach for healthcare practitioners Edited by Jo Haydon
© 2007 John Wiley & Sons, Ltd

The cell nucleus contains the chromosomes which carry the hereditary material, DNA, which is often referred to as the blueprint of the cell. This is because all the information for the production and function of any organism is contained within its DNA. A human fertilised egg or zygote contains DNA coding for all of the 23,000 genes.

The majority of normal cells are diploid, which means that they contain two sets of DNA, one derived from the maternal egg and the other from the paternal sperm. The exception to this is in males, where only one set of DNA from the X chromosome and one set of DNA from the Y chromosome is found. Genes are the templates for the production of the messenger RNA (mRNA) which carries the genetic information into the cytoplasm, where it is translated in order to produce a specific protein.

In order to pass only 23 chromosomes onto any potential offspring, the gametes (egg or sperm) must undergo a reduction division so that their chromosome number, and hence their DNA content, is halved. The result is called a haploid cell and the process whereby gametes (sperm and ova) are produced is termed meiosis.

CELL DIFFERENTIATION

In humans, many of the cells are differentiated, which means that they no longer have the capacity to perform all of the complex functions carried out by the whole organism. Differentiated cells are specialist cells capable of performing a unique function. For example, skeletal muscle cells contain a network of filaments made from proteins which can expand and contract; red blood cells become smooth sacks of haemoglobin which carry oxygen to the tissues.

Stem cells are cells which have not yet become differentiated. Embryonic stem cells have a greater capacity for following different pathways of differentiation than adult stem cells. The development of an embryo involves the production of many different cell types from unspecialised stem cells. Prior to differentiation, a stem cell can still divide and renew itself, and it can be persuaded to commit to differentiation along a specific pathway. During development, the position of the cell within the embryo and the signals each cell receives determine which cells become muscle cells and which become brain cells. Many specialised cells, such as nerve and heart cells cannot grow or divide, therefore they cannot repair tissue once it has become damaged.

CHROMOSOMES

Chromosomes are rod-like structures which carry the genes.

HISTORY

The normal number of human chromosomes was not recognised as 46 until 1956. Recognition of the first chromosomal disorder, Down syndrome, followed swiftly in 1959. In 1966, the Denver classification set the precedent for karyotyping or classifying human chromosomes. At that time chromosomes could only be solid stained so were sorted into groups according to their size and the position of the centromere, a constriction of the chromosome which separates it into two parts.

In 1971 Caspersson, a Swedish cytogeneticist and his team revolutionised the science of cytogenetics when they discovered a technique by which chromosomes could be stained to show a distinctive banding pattern. Each chromosome pair had its own unique pattern which distinguished it from all of the others. This permitted each pair to be defined and any abnormalities to be described with far greater accuracy. Now that each pair could be identified, the old group nomenclature was dropped and each chromosome pair was given a number, although the sex chromosomes remained as X and Y.

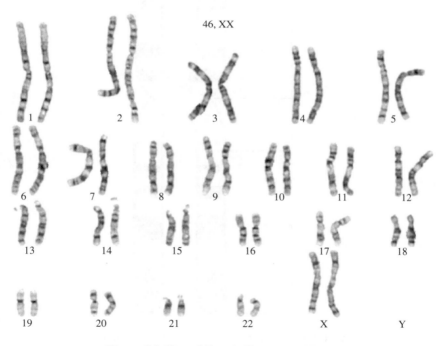

Figure 3.2 Normal Female Karyotype, 46, XX

In order to define chromosome abnormalities, it was necessary to number each of the bands along the chromosome arms. The bands are numbered starting at the centromere and out towards the chromosome tip. The major bands were first used to divide the chromosome arms into regions, and then individual bands both pale and dark were numbered within a region. So 1p21 means chromosome 1, short arm (p), region 2, band 1. A good quality karyotype, using Giesma staining, will have upwards of 800 bands, allowing the detection of even small abnormalities. As cytogenetics advanced and banding improved, producing even more bands per chromosome, it became necessary to subdivide them, so 1p21.2 now implies chromosome 1, short arm, region 2, band 1, sub-band 2.

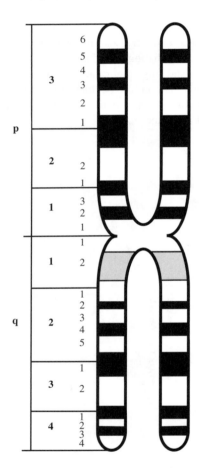

Figure 3.3 Banding Patterns on Human Chromosomes

We now know that the normal, or diploid, number of chromosomes in humans consists of 22 pairs of autosomes and one pair of sex chromosomes. The autosomal chromosomes are numbered according to size, with the largest designated pair numbered 1 and the smallest pair numbered 22, plus the two sex chromosomes,

X and Y. One of each of the autosomal pairs and one of the sex chromosomes is inherited from each parent.

- Females have the karyotype 46, XX; 44 autosomes and two copies of the X chromosome. They therefore have two copies of the genes found on the X chromosome. A female always passes on one of her X chromosomes to her offspring.
- Males have the karyotype 46, XY; 44 autosomes, an X and a Y chromosome. They therefore only have one copy of the genes found on the X chromosome and one copy of the male determining genes found on the Y chromosome. A male can pass on either his X or his Y chromosome to his offspring. It is the father who determines the sex of a child as passing on the X results in a female and passing on the Y results in a male.

The majority of chromosomes in the human karyotype have the centromere displaced from the middle, so that they have both a short and a long arm; such chromosomes are known as sub-metacentric. The short arm is called 'p' (from French *petit*) and the long arm is called 'q'. Convention still dictates that all chromosomes are aligned in the karyotype with the p arm at the top, above the centromere, and the q arm at the bottom. Some human chromosomes have the centromere approximately in the centre so that either side of it the two arms are of equal length, as in chromosomes 1, 3, 16, 19 and 20; they are termed metacentric. Others have the centromere positioned so that the short arm is very small and the genes are almost entirely located on the long arm. These are termed acrocentric chromosomes. Chromosomes 13, 14, 15, 21 and 22 are acrocentric.

In a modern diagnostic laboratory, chromosomes are studied by fluorescence *in situ* hybridisation, or FISH. This is a combination of cytogenetic and molecular techniques. The chromosomes are denatured, or made single stranded, while still on the slide, and are then treated with a fluorescent probe, which is complementary to a specific region of the genome. This enables cytogeneticists to identify the micro deletion syndromes, such as William's or Angelman's syndromes, in which a small amount of chromosomal material becomes lost or deleted from a particular location. Probes made from whole chromosomes, commonly called chromosome paints, can be used to detect submicroscopic translocations, as individual chromosomes can be painted with differently coloured fluorescent reporter molecules. This method also allows the identification of small additional marker chromosomes.

CELL DIVISION: MITOSIS AND MEIOSIS

MITOSIS

The cell cycle can be divided into a resting phase, known as interphase, and a phase of normal cell division, called mitosis. Mitosis is responsible for body growth and repair of damaged tissues. At mitosis, the chromosomes are copied and distributed into two daughter cells, each of which has exactly the same set of chromosomes as the original parent cell.

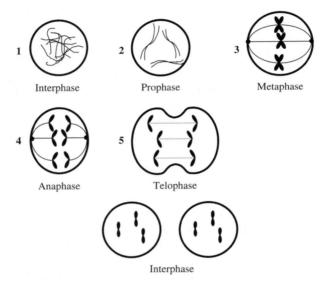

Figure 3.4 Cell Cycle Showing Interphase and Mitosis

Interphase is divided into stages called:

- G1: molecules are synthesised.
- S: DNA is copied.
- G2: manufacture of the membranes that will surround the daughter cells after division occurs.

Mitosis is divided into stages called:

- Prophase: the nuclear membrane breaks down and the chromosomes condense. Each chromosome now consists of two identical halves, called chromatids, which are joined at the centromere.
- Metaphase: the chromosomes are at their shortest and are now visible down the microscope.
- Anaphase: the chromosomes split in half vertically and the chromatids are pulled apart, one of each going into both of the new daughter cells.
- Telophase: the nuclear membrane reforms, the cell membrane divides and there are now two nuclei, each containing identical chromosome material located within a new daughter cell.

MEIOSIS

Our somatic or body cells undergo mitosis, while our reproductive cells undergo meiosis, a different type of cell division. The outcome here is not two identical daughter cells but individual gametes, each of which is haploid, containing only 23 chromosomes.

- Meiosis I: the nucleus doubles its DNA. Then each pair of chromosomes joins along their whole length. They are so closely joined that they can exchange material by crossing over, or 'recombination'. This causes the maternally and paternally inherited genes to become mixed, so each individual person has a mixture of their grandparental DNA, rather than inheriting an unchanged copy of the parental chromosome. This ensures a variation in inheritance patterns of genes instead of a continued passage of the same alleles (alternative forms of the same gene) each time. This is one of the reasons why siblings sometimes do not seem to be very alike. After this exchange of material, the chromosomes lie opposite each other on the spindle, and at anaphase they all move, each going in a different direction so that one of each pair goes into each daughter cell. This is the reduction division and each daughter cell contains only 23 chromosomes, one from each pair.

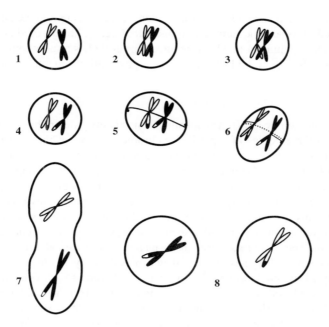

Figure 3.5 Meiosis I

- Meiosis II: essentially the same as a mitotic division, with the chromosomes lining up on a spindle by their centromeres and the chromatids separating vertically, but meiosis II takes place with 23, not 46 chromosomes. The X and the Y also pair together at meoisis and exchange material, but they only join and recombine at the short arm of the Y chromosome and the tip of the short arm of the X chromosome, so they meet in a 'head on' position rather than combining along their lengths. In males, the final result of meiosis is the production of four haploid gametes or sperm. At meiosis I, two secondary spermatocytes are formed, which at meiosis II divide to form two spermatids. These then develop into spermatozoa. So each primary spermatocyte produces four haploid sperm. The egg, or ovum, however, is much larger than the sperm and needs to retain cytoplasmic organelles such as mitochondria. In order to achieve this, the primary oocyte does not divide equally but produces one secondary oocyte and a small polar body which contains one of the haploid genomes. At meiosis II the same occurs; the secondary oocyte divides to form an ovum or egg cell and another polar body. So only a single ovum results from each female primary oocyte and all of the available cytoplasm and cytoplasmic bodies are concentrated into this single large cell.

CHROMOSOMAL ABNORMALITIES

A cell with a normal chromosome complement is called a euploid cell, and one with an abnormal chromosome number, an aneuploid cell. Chromosome anomalies are classified both by number and by structure. Very little has to go wrong with human chromosomes before individuals are affected physically or mentally, or both.

NUMERICAL ABNORMALITIES

The most common type of chromosomal abnormality is a trisomy, in which the cells contain three copies of a particular chromosome rather than the normal two. Trisomy arises at meiosis. Either a chromosome pair (at meiosis I) or the two chromatids (at meiosis II) fail to separate and one daughter cell acquires two copies, while the other receives none at all. Fertilisation of such a disomic gamete leads to a trisomic foetus. Monosomy of an autosome chromosome is invariably lethal, so is not seen. This main mechanism for the production of trisomies or abnormalities of chromosome number is non-disjunction at meiosis, which occurs more in the ovum than the sperm and increases in frequency with maternal age.

Most autosomal trisomies are lethal and usually only trisomy 13, trisomy 18 and trisomy 21 are compatible with live birth. Individuals with these trisomies are severely affected both physically and mentally; the effects are described in more detail in Chapter 6. Most autosomal trisomic foetuses abort spontaneously in the first trimester of pregnancy. More than half of such spontaneous losses tend to be chromosomally abnormal.

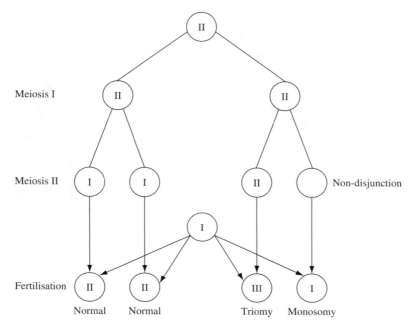

Figure 3.6 Non-Disjunction of a Pair of Chromosomes and Outcome Following Fertilisation

MOSAICISM

This usually occurs following normal fertilisation. At some stage in early embryonic life, non-disjunction occurs at mitosis in some cells. This results in one line of trisomy cells alongside a second line of normal cells and the degree of effect may be less severe than with non-disjunction at meiosis (see Figure 3.7). The earlier after fertilisation the non-disjunction occurs, the greater the percentage of trisomic cells and the greater the effect upon the individual.

STRUCTURAL ABNORMALITIES

Sometimes there is a trisomy or monosomy of only part of a chromosome rather than the whole of it. This can often occur as the result of an unbalanced reciprocal translocation or through production of a marker chromosome. A translocation occurs when two non-homologous chromosomes (i.e. chromosomes not from the same pair) break and, instead of rejoining correctly, exchange material, resulting in two rearranged chromosomes (see Chapter 6). If there is no loss or gain of DNA in such a reciprocal translocation, it is said to be balanced and the recipient is usually clinically unaffected. However, he or she is at risk of passing on the translocation in unbalanced form, resulting in miscarriage, reduced fertility or chromosomally abnormal offspring. Although individuals who carry translocations in a balanced

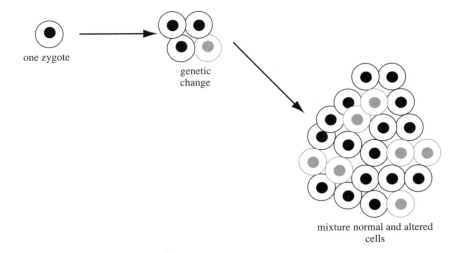

Figure 3.7 Mosaicism

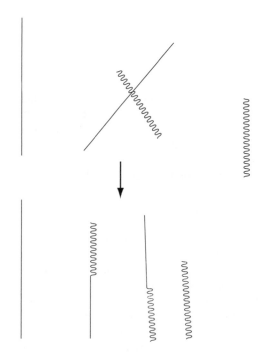

Figure 3.8 Breakage and Realignment of Chromosomes to Form a Reciprocal Translocation

form will most probably be unaffected, this is one of the rare chromosomal anomalies that can run in families, with some members inheriting it in an unbalanced form, often with severe consequences.

A variation on trisomy 21 which accounts for about 5% of individuals with Down syndrome is the result of a different type of translocation, termed a Robertsonian translocation, in which two acrocentric chromosomes become fused head to head at the centromere. Both short arms are lost but the material that they contain is repetitive, so there is no detrimental effect. Although a Robertsonian translocation can occur between any two acrocentric chromosomes, the most common type involves chromosomes 14 and 21. If the translocation is balanced then the carrier will have the karyotype 45, t(14;21) –14, –21 and be unaffected. If he or she passes on both the translocated 14;21 chromosome and a further copy of chromosome 21 then the child will have the karyotype 46, t(14;21) +21 and will have Down syndrome.

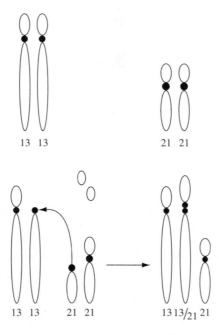

Figure 3.9 Breakage and Realignment of Chromosomes to Form a Robertsonian Translocation

Deletions, duplications, inversions and marker chromosomes can occur when chromosome breakages are repaired incorrectly. Deletions occur when a part of a chromosome is lost; duplications and insertions involve a gain of chromosomal material; and inversions are the result of a single chromosome suffering two breaks and the material in between them turning around before repair. Even when small segments of chromosomes are duplicated or deleted the effect on the individual can be very severe.

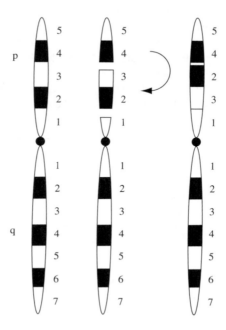

Figure 3.10 Chromosome Inversion

As with whole chromosomes, gain of part of the chromosome material is not as severe as loss of part of the material. Monosomy, or loss of material, for very small areas of the autosomes causes a series of syndromes known as the micro deletion syndromes, in which a very small deletion is present. For each particular syndrome, these deletions occur at very specific loci. They cannot always be detected by routine cytogenetic means so fluorescence *in situ* hybridisation (FISH) is employed. The micro deletion can be detected by using a specific fluorescent DNA probe from the deleted region. If the probe does not hybridise, or 'stick', to the specific region then a deletion must be present.

X AND Y CHROMOSOME ANOMALIES

The lack of effect that an extra copy of the Y chromosome exerts can be explained by the fact that the Y chromosome carries very few genes. Genes that are linked to the Y are either involved in male determination, such as the SRY gene, or tend to have an equivalent copy on the X chromosome. Much of the long arm of the Y chromosome consists of highly repetitive DNA, or heterochromatin, which does not contain functioning genes. The male determining genes are believed to imprint maleness upon a basic female, which explains why people with Turner syndrome are girls even though they could have lost either an X or a Y chromosome.

So why does the presence of an extra copy of the larger and gene-rich X chromosome not exert more of an effect? The explanation lies in the fact that humans cannot tolerate even small imbalances in their chromosomal material. This being so, how could we tolerate half of the population (female) having two copies of an average-sized chromosome with many genes, while the other half of the population (male) has only one copy? Surely this cannot be compensated for by a small chromosome with a marked lack of functioning genes? In fact, we do not tolerate this state of affairs, and every normal female is a mosaic. Very early in embryogenesis, every cell in a female embryo makes the independent and random decision to switch off (inactivate or Lyonise) one of her two X chromosomes. Because the process is random, half of her cells will have the maternally inherited X chromosome remaining active and the other half will have the paternally inherited X chromosome remaining active, hence she is a mosaic. The result is that dosage compensation is achieved and the two halves of the population have approximately equal numbers of active genes. The genes at the tip of the short arm of the X chromosome, at Xp22.3, where it exchanges with the Y chromosome at meiosis, do not inactivate and they constitute the pseudo autosomal region (PAR).

Females do not suffer from X-linked diseases such as haemophilia because, even if they are carriers of such a disorder, the half of their cells carrying the normal X chromosome will provide them with sufficient gene product for them to remain unaffected. On first describing X-inactivation in 1961, Mary Lyon found that once an X chromosome had been selected for inactivation it remained inactive throughout cell division, so that all progeny of the original cell had the same X inactive. An X chromosome only becomes reactivated during production of the reproductive cells or gametes.

Although even small abnormalities in the autosomes exert a very severe effect upon the individual unlucky enough to carry them, the same is not true of the sex chromosomes. Turner syndrome 45, X0 is the only non-lethal occurrence of monosomy of a whole chromosome.

Sex Chromosome Abnormalities

- Turner syndrome 45, X0.
- Klinefelter syndrome 47, XXY.
- Triple X syndrome 47, XXX.
- Male syndrome 47, XYY.

These syndromes can also exist in mosaic form, where there is a corresponding alleviation of symptoms. They are discussed in more detail in Chapter 6.

DNA: DEOXYRIBONUCLEIC ACID

Think of the structure and organisation of DNA as an individual's book, or blueprint, which comes in two volumes – one from the mother and one from the father.

Table 3.1 Individual's book – DNA

Book	Individual's DNA
Chapters	Chromosomes
Sentences (informative/descriptive)	Genes (exons/introns)
Words (3 letters: triplets or codons)	Amino Acids (building blocks of life)
Letters	Bases (A, C, G, T)

Like a book, it is divided into chapters, each one representing a chromosome.

The chapters are made up of sentences. Some of these are informative and essential; others are descriptive and may be superfluous.

The words within the sentences always contain three letters.

The DNA 'alphabet' only contains four letters.

We all have about 9 billion cells making up our bodies. Most of these cells, with the exception of the red blood cells, contain a nucleus. The nucleus carries the hereditary information stored in the form of deoxyribonucleic acid or DNA.

DNA exists in the form of a double helix, in which two separate strands are wound around each other in opposite directions. The main spiral of the double helix is made from a sugar-phosphate backbone and attached to each of the sugar rings is one of four different bases:

- Two purines, called adenine (A) and guanine (G).
- Two pyrimidines, called thymine (T) and cytosine (C).

Adenine always pairs with thymine and guanine always pairs with cytosine. The bases face inwards and hold the two strands together with weak bonds called hydrogen bonds. The hydrogen bonds are relatively weak so the two strands can be separated relatively easily without destroying the chain itself. The genetic information is coded by the sequence of bases in one DNA strand and the exactly complementary sequence on the other strand.

REPLICATION OF DNA

When a new DNA chain is made, the two strands of the DNA helix are separated and two new strands are assembled by copying the sequence of bases on each of the originals. DNA can only contain A=T and G=C, and this is the basis for exact duplication of the original strand. Thus:

- If adenine occurs on the original chain then a thymine must be put into the new chain.

- If thymine occurs on the original chain then an adenine must be put into the new chain.
- If guanine occurs on the original chain then a cytosine must be put into the new chain.
- If cytosine occurs on the original chain then a guanine must be put into the new chain.

So the new strand is an exact copy of one of the original strands. The base pairing of the sequence on one chain predetermines the sequence of the other. As the sequence on one chain is compatible only with a particular sequence on the other one, the two chains are said to be complementary. The enzyme which replicates the strands is called DNA polymerase. As both of the original strands act as templates for the production of the new ones, the result is two new double helices, each of which is an exact replica of the original one, and each of which contains one of the original strands and one newly replicated one. So each daughter cell has exactly the same DNA content and therefore exactly the same genetic information as the parent cell. Each receives one old chain from the original DNA molecule and one newly copied chain; this is called semi-conservative replication.

GENES

Genes are discrete sequences of DNA that can code for the amino-acid sequences of proteins. The information is encoded on the template strand of the continuous DNA double helical molecule. The DNA stores the genetic information and directs the synthesis of RNA (ribonucleic acid) molecules during transcription.

The DNA in the nuclear genome is arranged into genes, which are contained within the chromosomes. The human genome has 3000 million base pairs of DNA and about 23,000 genes. There is much too much DNA to code for just 23,000 genes. So interspersed in coding information are large stretches of DNA that have no coding function. Much of this is highly repetitive. About 80–90% of our genome comprises non-coding DNA, of which about 50% is repetitive.

Most of our genes are not continuous but are made up of small pieces called exons, with larger introns in between them. The exons are the coding sequences and the introns are intervening or non-coding sequences.

Human genes vary in size from the very small, about 100 base pairs, to the very large. The gene for Duchenne muscular dystrophy is about 2.4 million base pairs long and contains 70 exons.

TRANSCRIPTION

This is the process by which the information held in the DNA molecule within the cell nucleus is transferred (transcribed) into the intermediary ribonucleic acid molecule. During this process, the base thymine is replaced by uracil (U). Genes need to be transcribed in order to be active. Transcription is the copying of the DNA sequence of a gene into an equivalent sequence of RNA.

When the entire genomic sequence has been copied into RNA, the introns are cut out (spliced), leaving only the exons. This modified RNA is known as messenger RNA (mRNA). When it leaves the nucleus and enters the cytoplasm of the cell it can be translated into an amino acid sequence using the genetic or triplet code. Within the ribosomes, the amino acids are joined together to make the proteins.

TRANSLATION

Transcription is the production of RNA using DNA as a template. Translation is the assembly of amino acids into a protein chain using mRNA as a template. The genetic code is translated into a sequence of amino acids, which form a protein. Bases are read three at a time, with no punctuation. Each of these triplets, known as codons, specifies a particular amino acid. The triplet codons and the amino acids that they specify are termed 'the genetic code'.

There are 20 essential amino acids and only four bases. There are 64 possible combinations of the four bases into triplet codes.

Codons	Amino Acids
GCG, GCC, GCG, GCU	Alanine
AGA, AGG, CGA, CGC, CGG, CGU	Arginine
GAC, GAU	Aspartic acid
AAC, AAU	Asparagine
UGC, UGU	Cysteine
GAA, GAG	Glutamine acid
CAA, CAG	Glutamine
GGA, GGC, GGG, GGU	Glycine
CAC, CAU	Histidine
AUA, AUC, AUU	Isoleucine
UUA, UUG, CUA, CUC, CUG, CUU	Leucine
AAA, AAG	Lysine
AUG	Methionine
UUC, UUU	Phenylalanine
CGA, CCC, CCG, CCU	Proline
AGC, AGU, UCA, UCG, UCU	Serine
ACA, ACC, ACG, ACU	Threonine
UGG	Tryptophan
UAC, UAU	Tyrosine
GUA, GUC, GUG, GUU	Valine
UAA, UAG, UGA	STOP

Figure 3.11 Codons and Amino Acids

The genetic code therefore has more than one triplet coding for nearly every amino acid. The exceptions to this are methionine and tryptophan, which each have only one triplet coding for them. The codons UAA, UAG and UGA do not code for amino acids and are called nonsense codons. More correctly, they should be termed stop codons as they specify the end of the 'reading frame' or coded message of the mRNA molecule.

The sequence of bases along a DNA strand provides the information specifying the order of the amino acids along a polypeptide chain which will produce a specific protein.

ALTERATIONS IN DNA

Mutations

Our genetic information is stored as DNA, which is faithfully copied when it is replicated. RNA is an exact copy of the genes coded by the DNA – so can our genes ever alter?

Despite the exact replication and a built-in detect-and-repair mechanism, mistakes sometimes occur during DNA replication which can cause changes in the DNA sequence of a gene.

Mutations (changes) in genes can result in the production of abnormal proteins. This is the basis for many genetic diseases, so generally mutations are harmful, but if there were never any changes in DNA there would be no evolution. A mutation is a change in DNA or an alteration in the genotype. If there is a corresponding change in the expression of the gene, this is called a mutant phenotype.

A mutation can either occur spontaneously or it can be induced. Mutagens are chemicals or radiation that increases the mutation rates of genes. Different human genes mutate at different rates, with the average mutation rate of a human gene being about 1 in 10^6/gene/generation.

- A germinal mutation arises during meiosis or gamete production and affects all of the cells of an individual who carries it.
- A somatic mutation arises during mitosis or normal cell division and will only affect some body cells; the progeny of the cell in which it has arisen. Somatic mutations are often associated with malignancy.

Let us consider how the DNA sequence may be altered. To illustrate these possible alterations, let us say that the normal gene should read 'get the cat off the mat'.

Deletion

When one base, one triplet or several triplets are lost, e.g.

- One letter (base): 'get the cao fft hem at' (also known as a point mutation).
- One word (triplet): 'get the cat the mat'.
- A phrase (several triplets): 'get the cat'.

Insertion

When one base, one triplet or several triplets are added, e.g.

- One letter (base): 'get the cat sof fth ema t' (also known as a point mutation).
- One word (triplet): 'get the cat off the red mat'.
- A phrase (several triplets): 'get the cat off the old wet red mat'.

Substitution

When one base is changed to another, e.g.

- 'Get the cat off she mat' (also known as a point mutation).
- 'Get the hat' (where hat = stop message).

Polymorphisms

These occur when alterations in the DNA sequence do not result in the alteration of a gene, or when they occur in the non-coding regions. Alterations in one letter (point mutations) may have no effect on the gene product, as we have seen that most of the amino acids have several triplets coding for them, e.g. GGA codes for glycine, but so too do GGG, GGC and GGU.

These types of change occur fairly frequently and are called SNPs or single nucleotide polymorphisms.

The deletion or insertion of bases in multiples of three (triplets), while leading to additional or missing amino acids, *may* have no effect on the structure of the protein produced. Polymorphisms contribute to the variability between individuals.

Types of Mutation

Alterations in the DNA sequence causing mutations can be divided into different types:

- Missense mutation, where one amino acid is replaced with another, e.g. 'get the rat off the mat'.
- Nonsense mutation, where a stop codon is introduced, e.g. 'get the hat'.
- Frameshift mutation, where deletion or insertion of one or two bases (but not three), or any number that is not a multiple of three, will alter the reading frame of the message, e.g. (deletion) 'get the cao fft hem at'; (insertion) 'get the cat sof fth ema t'. These are often lethal as, beyond the mutation, the codons will be completely incorrect.

DNA can become mutated by many different mechanisms, ranging from a single substitution of a base to a large-scale chromosomal disruption. Mutations at the level of the gene can be substitutions, additions, expansions, deletions or rearrangements. Substitution of a different amino acid, particularly one of a different type, can cause severe genetic disease. For example, a single base change in codon 6 of the β-globin gene from GAG to GTG (changing glutamic acid to valine) causes sickle cell anaemia. Severe deletions are not always associated with frameshifts; the deletion of the triplet CTT in codon 508 of the CFTR gene eliminates a phenylalanine and causes cystic fibrosis.

Chromosomal mutations can be of both number and structure, such as a trisomy or a translocation. In chronic myeloid leukaemia, the malignant cells demonstrate a translocation between chromosomes 9 and 22, which results in an apparently foreshortened chromosome 22, christened the Philadelphia (Ph') chromosome. In remission, the translocation is present in fewer cells. The presence of this small Philadelphia chromosome allows the progress of the disease to be monitored and aids in both the prognosis and decisions concerning the type of therapy which should be offered.

In human cells, nuclear DNA in chromosomes exists as chromatin. There are two types of chromatin, euchromatin, which contains the active genes, and heterochromatin, which is not transcribed.

GENOTYPE/PHENOTYPE CORRELATIONS

The central dogma of molecular biology is defined as DNA → RNA → PROTEIN.

The production of proteins from a gene is called gene expression. Some genes, such as the ribosomal (rRNA) genes or the transfer (tRNA) genes, do not have a protein product as they function as RNA. Certain others control other genes by switching them on or off.

The genotype of an individual is his or her genetic makeup. The phenotype is the result of this genetic makeup, or how the genes are expressed in the individual. The phenotype is the appearance of and properties displayed by the individual as a direct result of their genotype. If a mutation is detected in a human genome, the likely clinical effect upon the individual who carries it can be predicted. For example:

- An extra copy of chromosome 21 will result in Down syndrome.
- A missense mutation GAG → GTG in codon 6 of the haemoglobin gene (changing glutamic acid to valine) will cause sickle cell anaemia.
- The loss of CTT at codon 508 of the CFTR gene (ΔF508) will result in cystic fibrosis.

Once a mutation has been detected in a family and is confirmed as causing a disorder, those members who do not carry it can be reassured that they will not develop the disease. Those who do carry a mutant gene can be followed-up more carefully, particularly in cases of the germline mutations which predispose to malignancy, such as those which occur in the so-called 'breast cancer' genes BRCA1 and BRCA2.

MITOCHONDRIA

Almost all cells are powered by mitochondria. Each cell contains many of these organelles, which generate chemical energy by oxidising fats and sugars and produce adenosine tri-phosphate (ATP), which carries this energy within the phosphate bonds to wherever it is required. Not all the DNA in the cell is contained within the nucleus.

The mitochondrion carries its own DNA, which has slight variations. Mitochondrial DNA is circular and has no nuclear membrane bounding it. Mitochondria are inherited only from the egg, not from sperm, so there is only maternal inheritance of the genetic diseases resulting from mutations in the mitochondrial DNA.

POINTS FOR REFLECTION

- There are 3 billion (3,000,000,000) letters in the DNA code in every cell in your body.
- There is 1.8 m of DNA in each of our cells, packed into a structure only 0.001 m across (it would easily fit on the head of a pin!).
- The vast majority of DNA in the human (97%) has no known function.
- Our DNA is 98% identical to chimpanzees'.
- Between humans, DNA differs by only 0.2%.

4 Laboratory Techniques

EILEEN ROBERTS AND SARAH WARBURTON

CYTOGENETICS

Cytogenetics is the study of chromosomes. Molecular genetics (often referred to as 'DNA technology') involves the study of the genetic material at the level of the individual nucleotide bases that make up DNA.

OBTAINING METAPHASE CELLS FOR ANALYSIS

Conventional cytogenetic study of human chromosomes generally requires cells to be in a state of division. The most straightforward tissue to study is blood, in which the nucleated cells are the lymphocytes. Circulating lymphocytes are not usually found in a dividing state in healthy individuals and need to be cultured to stimulate cell division, through the addition of a mitogen. Addition of a mitogen provokes an antigenic response, which in human lymphocytes results in waves of mitotic activity, commencing after an initial lag of 30 hours or so. Short-term lymphocyte cultures can be harvested (see later) after 48, 72 or 96 hours.

Cells derived from other sources, e.g. amniotic fluid cells obtained at amniocentesis and solid tissue biopsies, need to be encouraged to enter cell division by being cultured (long-term culture) in sterile conditions, in an environment which provides all the necessary conditions (nutrients, temperature, pH) for active cell growth. The introduction of contaminants (bacteria, fungi) into long-term culture, either by contamination at sampling or during cell culture, is extremely detrimental to cell growth and will in most cases lead to culture failure. It is therefore essential that scrupulous procedures for control of infection are maintained at all stages, from taking the sample to harvesting the culture.

In long-term culture, the length of time taken to achieve sufficient cell growth to allow chromosome analysis to be performed varies with tissue type and culture medium. For amniotic fluid cells, culture times range from 7–20 days (UK average for the period 2001–2: 13 days; UKNEQAS data). The range for other tissue types can be much wider. Each individual patient sample will have its own unique set of growth dynamics and therefore, while most samples will grow within a predictable

Genetics in Practice: A clinical approach for healthcare practitioners   Edited by Jo Haydon
© 2007 John Wiley & Sons, Ltd

range of culture times, it is impossible to accurately define culture times for samples on an individual basis. This can sometimes present anxiety in prenatal diagnosis samples, as patients are faced with a somewhat indeterminate wait for their results, dependent on the growth dynamics of their individual sample.

In order to obtain chromosome preparations from cells after short or long-term culture, the cultures are subjected to a harvesting procedure. In culture, the cells undergo mitosis; in order to visualise the chromosomes, the cells are blocked during the metaphase stage (see Chapter 3).

At metaphase, chromosomes have contracted from their long tangled state to form identifiable structures. Various techniques exist for the synchronisation of cell cultures, the purpose of which is twofold: 1) to maximise the number of metaphase figures available at the time of harvest, and 2) to allow for a level of control over the length of the chromosomes. As the chromosomes proceed through cell division they contract, and the aim in harvesting is to achieve the optimal balance between chromosomes too long and tangled to analyse, and those too short to allow any great degree of detail to be visualised. Cultures are blocked at metaphase by the addition of an agent that prevents the formation of the mitotic spindle apparatus in cell division.

Following the blocking step, the cultures are exposed to hypotonic treatment to swell the cells. They are then fixed, using an acid/alcohol fixative. Fixed cell suspensions are dropped onto clean glass slides, thereby fracturing the cellular membranes and releasing the nuclei. As the cell suspensions dry on the slide, the nuclear membranes dissolve, leaving the chromosome preparations ready for analysis.

CHROMOSOME ANALYSIS

Standard Chromosome Analysis

In the UK, standard chromosome analysis is performed on G-banded preparations. Prepared slides undergo a series of enzymatic and chemical pre-treatments, followed by staining with Giemsa or similar stain (hence the name 'G-banding'). This results in each pair of chromosomes displaying a unique banding pattern, which allows them to be identified and paired. Any deviations from the pattern indicating a possible abnormality can be recognised.

Chromosome analysis is then performed, usually directly through a high-powered light microscope, although sometimes a karyotype will be produced using digital image enhancement software. The ability to analyse chromosome banding patterns is a precise skill requiring intensive training.

The first step in analysing chromosomes is to determine the count. Normal individuals have 46 chromosomes, comprising 22 homologous pairs of autosomes and two sex chromosomes, XX in females and XY in males.

Numerical chromosome anomalies (extra or missing chromosomes) are termed aneuploidies (see Chapter 6). The most common aneuploidies of the autosomes include trisomy (three copies) of chromosome 21 (Down syndrome), trisomy 18

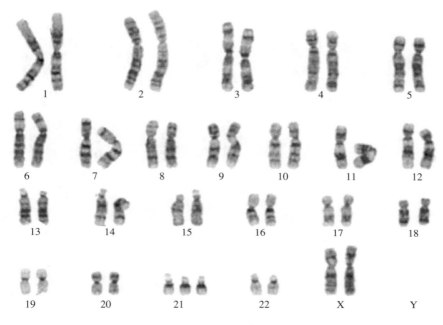

Figure 4.1 Female Trisomy 21 (Down Syndrome) Karyotype

(Edwards' syndrome) and trisomy 13 (Patau's syndrome). Aneuploidies of the sex chromosomes include conditions such as Turner syndrome, associated with the presence of monosomy (single) X chromosome in females (45, X karyotype), and Klinefelter syndrome in males, with the presence of an additional X chromosome (47, XXY karyotype). Occasionally, additional (usually small) unidentified marker chromosomes are detected; these are termed marker chromosomes when their origin is unknown.

The next step in chromosome analysis is a detailed band-by-band comparison of each individual homologue of the chromosome pairs. This may detect alterations in the banding pattern, which can be further characterised and identified, as each chromosome has its own unique pattern of bands. Structural chromosome rearrangements include translocations, in which parts of two different chromosomes exchange places. These may be balanced, when there is no loss or gain of genetic material, or unbalanced, when there is loss and/or gain of genetic material. Translocations may be inherited from one of the parents or may arise *de novo* (as a new event).

Other structural chromosome rearrangements include deletions of chromosome material (a microscopically visible deletion almost invariably being associated with phenotypic consequences such as congenital anomalies and learning difficulties in the individual carrying it) and inversions, in which a segment within a chromosome has been inverted relative to the rest of the chromosome.

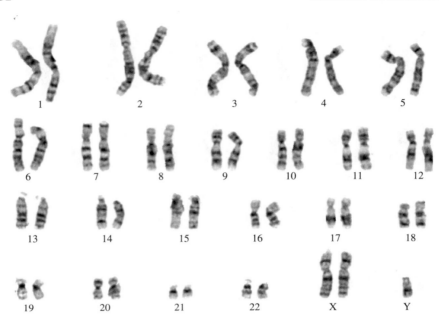

Figure 4.2 Klinefelter Syndrome XXY

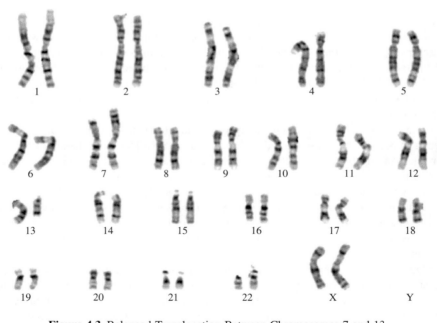

Figure 4.3 Balanced Translocation Between Chromosomes 7 and 13

Chromosome variants are alterations in the G-banding pattern which are inherited as familial variations of no consequence to the phenotype. Variants not previously recognised may present problems, especially at prenatal diagnosis, and can be characterised by a range of specialised staining techniques and FISH, which may be used to discriminate between material containing active genes (euchromatin) and genetically inert material (heterochromatin).

Fluorescence *In Situ* Hybridisation (FISH)

The reproducible pattern of chromosome bands described above can only be produced in metaphase chromosomes and therefore requires actively dividing cells. In addition, the resolution that can be achieved by G-banded analysis of metaphase chromosomes using a light microscope will only allow the identification of chromosome changes of 4 Mb or greater. In poorer quality preparations the level of resolution is lower still. In practice, this means that small rearrangements or changes in the chromosomes may not be detected by conventional cytogenetic analysis. Some microdeletions are not visible even at the highest resolutions of G-banded analysis.

FISH is a technique in which specific DNA probes (single-stranded pieces of DNA) detect their complementary sequences within the genome. This technique can be applied to non-dividing as well as dividing cells and therefore can be used in situations in which it is not possible to look at G-banded preparations.

The FISH technique takes a cloned piece of the genome with a reporter molecule attached. The probe is then allowed to hybridise (attach) to its complementary region within the chromosome, i.e. it hybridises *in situ*. A fluorescent reagent that binds to the reporter molecule attached to the DNA probe then identifies the location of this hybridisation. The fluorescence can be visualised using a microscope with special filter sets that detect light of different wavelengths. This visualisation allows the presence or absence of the sequence of interest to be determined, and for the specific chromosomal location to be determined in metaphase chromosomes. The FISH technique can be used to simultaneously detect the presence of several regions of interest, by the use of different fluorochromes (molecules which fluoresce when excited by light of a specific wavelength).

Applications of FISH

FISH is not dependent on the presence of dividing cells. It can therefore be used to determine the number of copies of a given sequence in interphase cells. For example, a probe specific to the Down syndrome 'critical region' on chromosome 21 has found wide application in the rapid detection of Down syndrome in uncultured amniotic fluid cells obtained at amniocentesis. This allows a rapid result to be issued and, for many patients, relieves the considerable anxiety associated with the wait for results from cultured cells.

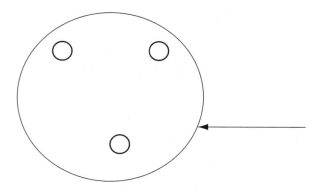

Figure 4.4 Interphase Cell Showing Three Copies of Chromosome 21 Specific Probe

FISH can be used to determine the presence or absence of a specific sequence of interest. For example, the majority of cases of DiGeorge syndrome, which is associated with cardiac defects, absent or defective thymus, cleft palates and often other malformations, are caused by a sub-microscopic deletion within chromosome 22 at band q11.2. Before the advent of FISH technology this deletion was largely unknown. However, the development of a molecular probe specific to this region has allowed a diagnostic test to be developed which can be applied to all suspected cases to confirm the diagnosis.

Marker chromosomes and other structural chromosome rearrangements can be investigated by FISH. Chromosome paints consist of a collection of DNA probes which hybridise along the length of a specific chromosome and are all linked to the same fluorochrome, such that under fluorescence microscopy in metaphase cells, the whole chromosome is 'painted' with the appropriate colour fluorescence. This allows for the identification of marker chromosomes, which in turn can aid in prognostic information; it can also be used as a tool in characterising translocations and other rearrangements, where different chromosomes are painted with different fluorochromes.

A recent development of the FISH technique has been its use in determining changes involving the subtelomeric sequences, regions at the ends of the chromosomes which may be involved in rearrangements that are beyond the resolution of conventional microscopy, and which have been implicated particularly in idiopathic mental retardation.

FISH Technique

FISH is performed on fixed cells, either on metaphase preparations obtained as above, or on fixed uncultured cells dropped onto glass slides. It is also possible to perform FISH on fixed paraffin sections.

Preparation may include pre-treatment steps to increase permeability of the cells to the probe. The probe and target DNA are then treated to denature them (make them single-stranded), so that they will be able to adhere to one another. They are then co-hybridised, usually at 37 °C to allow for the most efficient hybridisation. The preparations are treated by washing to remove any unbound probe or probe loosely attached to non-complementary DNA. These stringency washes are designed to remove any probe which is not securely attached to its complementary sequence (i.e. non-specific binding), while leaving the matched probe-target complex intact. The bound probe and target can be visualised directly under the appropriate wavelength fluorescence if the probe was directly attached to a fluorochrome, or indirectly after a detection step when the probe has a reporter molecule attached.

Comparative Genomic Hybridisation (CGH)

CGH (Kallioniemi *et al.*, 1992) is a technology that allows gains or losses of chromosomal material to be characterised, even from tissues from which it is not possible to obtain metaphase preparations, e.g. tumour tissue. The technique compares the DNA from the tissue/subject of interest (the 'test' DNA) to control or reference DNA. This is achieved by labelling the test DNA with a fluorochrome of one colour, e.g. red, and the reference DNA with a fluorochrome of a different colour, e.g. green. The two DNAs are then allowed to compete for sites of hybridisation on normal metaphase spreads; where the test and reference DNAs are present in a 1:1 ratio, neither colour will predominate, but where the 1:1 ratio is disturbed by gains or losses of DNA in the test material, either the red (gain) or green (loss) will predominate.

Sophisticated software is used to accurately determine the relative proportions of the test and reference DNA and produces a CGH profile, in which deviation from the 1:1 ratio appears as a shift from the median line.

CGH can therefore be used to determine imbalances anywhere in the genome. Its resolution for deletions lies between 5 and 20 Mb. It has many applications in tumour genetics, in which it is often difficult to obtain metaphase preparations, and in situations where only fixed or frozen tissue is available. However, note that it will not detect balanced chromosome rearrangements such as translocations and inversions; it is a technique for measuring relative copy number changes in test DNA.

MOLECULAR GENETICS

The use of techniques for analysing DNA, commonly referred to as molecular genetics, has only become recognisable as a diagnostic discipline in its own right in the last decade or so. The ability to analyse DNA has had an important impact on the understanding of genetic disorders. Many specific gene mutations have been identified, and a host of other genetic disorders, for which the genes are not yet

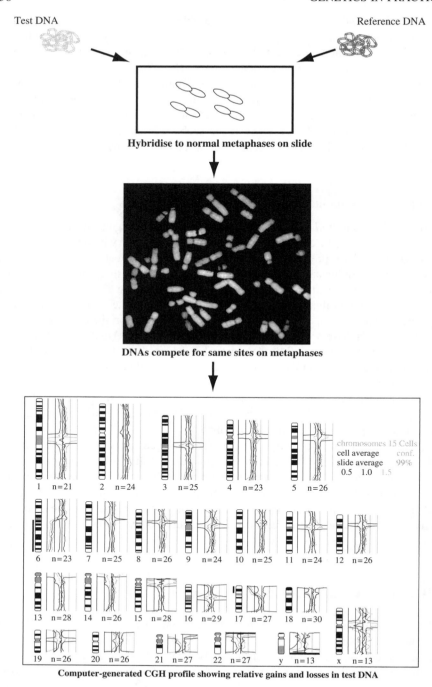

Test DNA

Reference DNA

Hybridise to normal metaphases on slide

DNAs compete for same sites on metaphases

chromosomes 15 Cells
cell average   conf.
slide average   99%
0.5   1.0   1.5

1   n=21   2   n=24   3   n=25   4   n=23   5   n=26

6   n=23   7   n=25   8   n=26   9   n=24   10   n=25   11   n=24   12   n=26

13   n=28   14   n=26   15   n=28   16   n=29   17   n=27   18   n=30

19   n=26   20   n=26   21   n=27   22   n=27   y   n=13   x   n=13

Computer-generated CGH profile showing relative gains and losses in test DNA

Figure 4.5 Comparative Genomic Hybridisation (Diagram supplied by Sara Dyer, Birmingham Women's Hospital NHS Trust.)

identified, have been mapped to particular chromosomal locations, which enables predictive testing using linked DNA markers.

The number of mapped genes is increasing at a high rate and there are now hundreds of identified DNA segments which may be used as markers for particular disorders. Many are clinically useful probes that can be applied to both detecting carriers and to prenatal diagnosis, as well as for confirmation of diagnoses in children and adults.

A molecular genetics diagnostic laboratory can perform various diagnostic procedures to determine if an individual is affected by a genetic disease. As a consequence, appropriate treatment can reduce the effects of, or even completely alleviate, any signs of the disease in question. This is especially important in prenatal diagnosis, where parents have the opportunity to receive extensive counselling and then come to a decision about the fate of their unborn child (see Chapter 5). Because chorionic villus sampling is performed at 11–12 weeks of gestation, investigating and counselling a family prior to pregnancy is important to ensuring that a couple has time to come to fully informed decisions.

As already mentioned, diagnosis of genetic disease often involves family studies. Families wish to know what the risks are to their relatives and may also wish to discuss the lifestyle options available to them.

METHODOLOGIES

DNA testing can essentially be split into two different approaches. The first involves testing for specific mutations that are known to be causative for a disease in all affected patients, and the second involves screening particular genes to look for changes in the DNA which can cause disease, but where the particular change involved tends to vary from family to family.

The techniques used to detect unknown mutations in a sample of DNA are relatively difficult and costly to perform, but where the mutation is known, simpler diagnostic methods are employed. Situations where this might be the case are:

- The mutation in one or more affected family members has been characterised and other family members require testing to know whether they are carriers of the condition.
- A common disease causing mutation is present at a high level in the general population, e.g. the delta F508 mutation responsible for cystic fibrosis.

The amount of information that can be provided by DNA tests depends on the current knowledge about the gene(s) involved and may be obtained in two ways:

- By direct testing: the patient's DNA is tested to determine whether a given pathogenic mutation is present.
- By indirect testing or gene tracking: linked markers are used in family studies to see whether or not the patient has inherited the disease-carrying chromosome.

Clearly, in general, direct testing is the approach of choice, but this is not always possible. The relevant gene must have been identified and the normal ('wild type') DNA sequence must be known. Direct testing is mostly done by polymerase chain reaction (PCR) technology, a technique which is extremely sensitive and allows the use of a wide range of sources of patient DNA, including:

- Blood samples: the most common source of adult DNA and that preferred by laboratories. It is important that blood samples for DNA extraction are received in EDTA collection tubes and that they are clearly and appropriately labelled with a minimum of two identifiers (e.g. name, date of birth) that match the information contained on the accompanying referral form.
- Mouthwash samples or buccal scrapes: sometimes used for population screening programmes or in cases where a patient is unwilling to provide a blood sample.
- Chorionic villus biopsy samples: the best source of foetal DNA for prenatal diagnosis.
- One or two cells removed from eight-cell stage embryos: for pre-implantation diagnosis following *in vitro* fertilisation.
- Guthrie cards: cards on which a spot of dried blood is preserved, generally taken from newborn infants.

On arrival at the laboratory, specimens are booked into a computerised patient database and everything that subsequently happens to a sample can be tracked via the computer records, up to and including the issue of a final report by the laboratory.

CATEGORIES OF DNA TEST

Molecular genetic testing may broadly be divided into four main categories, which are:

- Diagnostic testing.
- Carrier detection.
- Presymptomatic testing for adult onset diseases.
- prenatal diagnosis (PND).

Diagnostic Testing

Examples include testing to differentiate Huntington disease from other rare neurological disorders such as spinocerebellar ataxia; confirmation or exclusion of Fragile X syndrome as a cause of mental retardation; clarification of a diagnosis or suspicion of diseases such as cystic fibrosis, Prader-Willi syndrome, Angelman syndrome etc. This type of test is not always 100% reliable. For example, the failure to detect a dystrophin gene deletion in suspected cases of Duchenne or Becker muscular dystrophy does not exclude the diagnosis because in approximately 35% of affected individuals the mutation responsible is either a duplication or point mutation.

Carrier Detection Within Families

Such tests are relevant when, for example, a child has been diagnosed with congenital adrenal hyperplasia (CAH) caused by 21-hydroxylase deficiency and carrier detection is required for a sibling or other close blood relative. Molecular genetic testing can provide a powerful tool for this type of diagnosis and indeed may be the only method suitable for deriving carrier information.

Carrier Detection Within Populations

DNA testing for autosomal recessive diseases (i.e. where two copies of a gene mutation must be present for an individual to be affected) may not be the most efficient method of detecting carriers in populations. For diseases such as the haemoglobinopathies, carrier status can be determined on full blood count and red cell indices. However, for some diseases, such as cystic fibrosis, this is the only method available. Molecular genetics laboratories that undertake this sort of programme must have the resources to process relatively large numbers of referrals and have processing, analysis and reporting systems in place appropriate to the task. The fact that approximately 1 in 20 of the white British population are carriers of cystic fibrosis gives some indication of the scale of the task.

Any population screening programme must produce a useful outcome, such as neonatal screening for phenylketonuria, which enables appropriate treatment to be initiated promptly and greatly improves the prognosis for the patient.

Presymptomatic Testing

Presymptomatic testing for adult onset disorders requires that the mutation involved is recognised before such a test is available. For some disorders, e.g. Huntington disease, the mutation will always be the same (i.e. an expansion of the CAG triplet), whereas in other conditions, e.g. familial adenomatous polyposis (FAP) or breast/ovarian cancer, the mutation involved may vary from family to family. Close liaison between the laboratory and referring clinicians is necessary to ensure that the counselling protocols in place for such testing have been adhered to.

Prenatal Diagnosis (PND)

PND is often requested in order to detect severe childhood diseases where there is poor prognosis with little or no effective treatment. However, it is also requested for the detection of adult onset disorders, e.g. Huntington disease, myotonic dystrophy. The availability of accurate prenatal testing can have a dramatic impact on a couple's reproductive plans. Before the development of prenatal molecular tests, many parents of children with spinal muscular atrophy and cystic fibrosis chose not to have any further offspring. Many mothers/sisters/aunts/female cousins of boys with Duchenne muscular dystrophy wishing to prevent the possibility of having an affected son experienced the trauma of midtrimester termination of male foetuses.

Many couples with a family history of adult onset disorder remained childless, or if they did have children, felt fearful and guilty about the possibility of having passed on the altered gene. For many of these families, the option of PND has become a prerequisite for embarking on a pregnancy. Consequently, many healthy children have been born who would otherwise have been terminated, or would never been conceived, had PND not been possible.

For the molecular genetics laboratory, performing an urgent, complex test in pregnancy requires close collaboration with clinicians. Ideally, the required specimens should be obtained from the affected family member and from other family members prior to the requirement for PND. The laboratory then has the opportunity to perform the tests required in advance, for example, to make the family informative for a linkage based test or define the mutation involved. The actual prenatal test can then be carried out much faster.

Not all molecular genetic testing is used to detect inherited abnormalities. Increasingly, post-bone marrow transplant patients have their DNA tested to detect levels of host and donor stem cells. Testing is done regularly so that an increase in host stem cells, indicating a possible rejection of donor stem cells, can be detected and a suitable course of treatment initiated at an early stage to avoid relapse.

POLYMERASE CHAIN REACTION (PCR)

This technique is fundamental to the majority of methods used in DNA testing. It is a procedure that produces multiple copies of a specific short segment of DNA. The amplified stretch of DNA, doubled each cycle for 30 or so cycles, can then be subjected to further testing. PCR can amplify sequences from minute amounts of starting DNA, even from the DNA from a single cell. However, the extreme sensitivity of the technique means that great care must be taken to avoid contamination of the sample under investigation by external DNA, such as minute amounts of cells from the operator.

Quantitative Fluorescent PCR (QF-PCR)

QF-PCR analysis has recently entered the field of prenatal diagnosis to overcome the need to culture foetal cells and hence allow rapid diagnosis of certain selected chromosomal anomalies. It is used for the rapid detection of prenatal aneuploidy by a number of UK laboratories, the results being issued to clinical staff and followed up by a full karyotype analysis in all cases where cultures cells are available. Trisomies 13, 18 and 21 are routinely tested for and sex chromosome aneuploidy is investigated in a subset of referrals. The use of sex chromosome markers is decided in consultation with clinical colleagues.

For each chromosome tested, an abnormal result is reported when at least two of the markers used are consistent with a trisomic genotype. Mosaicism for trisomy and normal cell lines can be detected by QF-PCR and may be reported, though the clinical significance of such a result may be difficult to define. The QF-PCR sex chromosome assay is a stringent screen for monosomy X but is not a diagnostic test. A result where all X markers show only one peak and no Y sequences are present may represent a normal female homozygous for all markers used and thus a qualified report is issued.

By using QF-PCR as a stand-alone test, the chances of non-diagnosing the commonest chromosome anomalies, which increase in frequency with maternal age, are estimated to be 1 in 150 abnormal karyotypes, or 1 in 10–30,000 samples tested, depending on age distribution.

METHODS FOR DETECTING SPECIFIED MUTATIONS

Southern Blotting

This technique detects large deletions, expansions and rearrangements within DNA by digestion of genomic DNA with restriction endonuclease enzymes, followed by gel electrophoresis, transfer to artificial membrane and subsequent hybridisation with specific radiolabelled probes. The pattern of bound radioactivity is detected by autoradiography and mutations produce extra or different bands compared to normal. Fragile X is one disease that is investigated by this technique.

There are many other techniques for detecting the presence of known mutations, the details of which lie outside the scope of this book. They range from testing a gene for the presence of one or two specific mutations (e.g. testing for haemochromatosis) to testing for the presence of many different mutations within a gene. Over 1100 different mutations have so far been identified in the gene involved in cystic fibrosis and the number is still increasing! However, only 20 or so of these occur with any measurable frequency and laboratories routinely screen patients for the 31 most common mutations.

DNA Sequencing

Theoretically, direct sequencing of DNA can detect *all* changes in base sequence and thus all possible mutations within a gene. Fully automated sequencers are used, which produce computer print-outs of the DNA base sequence for both strands of the DNA under investigation and compare them with known normal controls. Mutations are fully characterised but this approach is laborious and generates excessive information. Direct sequencing is routinely used in the investigation of conditions such as breast cancer and von Hippel Lindau disease, and in all other diseases where different families generally carry different mutations.

Indirect Testing of DNA by Gene Tracking

Gene tracking was historically the first type of DNA diagnostic method to be widely used and the use of linked markers still has a place in modern molecular diagnosis. Necessities for successful linkage analysis are:

- To distinguish the two chromosomes of the parent(s) who may have transmitted the disease. Nowadays, with the availability of many highly informative DNA markers, this is generally quite straightforward.
- To establish phase, i.e. to work out which marker allele segregates with the disease allele.
- To find out which allele has been passed on to the affected individual and whether this is the same as that passed on to the family member being tested.

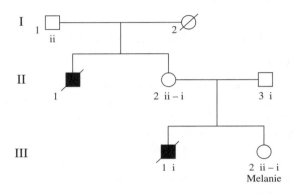

Figure 4.6 Pedigree Showing Linkage

In this pedigree representing X-linked inheritance, Melanie (III.3) is requesting testing as she wishes to know if she is a carrier of the gene alteration causing the disorder that has affected several males in her family. Her mother, II.2, has marker i and marker ii; she had inherited marker allele ii from her father and must therefore have inherited marker allele i from her mother, who was a carrier for this condition. Melanie has inherited allele i from her father and thus allele ii from her mother. Allele ii marks the unaffected X chromosome and thus the data suggests that Melanie is not a carrier of the disease.

Because the DNA marker sequence used for gene tracking is not the sequence that causes the disease, there is always the possibility of recombination between the disease and the marker. Recombination is the exchange of a segment of DNA between the chromosomes of a pair. The risk of recombination is minimised by using markers that lie as close as possible to the sequence that causes the disease.

Another potentially problematic aspect of gene tracking is the establishment of paternity. Non-paternity usually renders gene tracking impossible. It is important that the genetic team has a policy on what to do if non-paternity is discovered.

RECENT TECHNOLOGICAL ADVANCES: DENATURING HPLC

The development of new and more sophisticated techniques for the detection of mutations in genetic material is moving at a fast pace. Some recent advances include the introduction of pyrosequencing, TaqMan probe technology and oligonucleotide microarrays. It is beyond the scope of this chapter to describe these techniques in detail. One approach that has the potential for being used with huge numbers of samples for many different diseases, and which is already in use in many diagnostic laboratories, is WAVE technology. It is based on the fact that mutations and polymorphisms alter denaturing profiles of DNA. It allows detection of single base substitutions and small deletions or insertions in DNA fragments of up to 1500 bp in length.

The major advantages of dHPLC are its high sensitivity and specificity. A blind study of the blood clotting factor IX gene detected all 45 heterozygotes that were included in a total sample number of 93. The technique also enables a very rapid throughput of samples compared to other methods currently in use. With semi-automated analysis, samples take approximately six minutes to be processed. Although the initial cost of the equipment is high (about £75,000 per machine), subsequent running costs are cheap (about £1 per sample).

METABOLIC TESTS

Most inborn errors of metabolism follow autosomal recessive inheritance. A carrier of an autosomal recessive disorder is a healthy person who possesses the disease-causing mutation but also carries a normal copy of the gene which is sufficient for normal cell function (we call such a person a heterozygote). Heterozygotes may show reduced activities of specific enzymes, which can provide the basis for detecting carriers of the condition. The parents of an affected child are obligate carriers but testing may be needed for the healthy siblings of an affected person, and also for their partner if the condition is fairly common. Testing is also important for consanguineous couples with a family history of genetic disease. Biochemical identification of carriers may be possible when the gene product is known. This approach can be used for inborn errors of metabolism due to enzyme deficiency as well as for disorders caused by a defective structural protein, such as haemophilia and thalassaemia. When the gene product is not known or cannot be easily tested, carrier detection may depend on detecting secondary biochemical abnormalities, such as elevated serum creatine kinase in Duchenne and Becker muscular dystrophy.

In X-linked recessive disorders, parental carrier state is sometimes particularly difficult to assess due to the possibilities of a new mutation in the offspring or of germline mosaicism in the parent (see Chapter 9). However, these diseases are often severe and many female relatives may be at risk of having affected sons.

Biochemical tests designed to assess carrier status must be evaluated in obligate carriers from affected families. Only tests which give significantly different results in obligate carriers compared to normal controls are useful. Because ranges of values in obligate carriers and controls may overlap, such as with serum creatine kinase activity in X-linked Becker and Duchenne muscular dystrophy, problems may arise. Confirmation of carrier state is always easier than exclusion. In muscular dystrophy, a high serum creatine kinase activity confirms carrier status whereas a normal result reduces, but does not eliminate, the chance of a female being a carrier.

Obligate carriers do not always give abnormal biochemical values because of the phenomenon of lyonisation, i.e. the process by which one or other X chromosome in female embryonic cells is inactivated early in embryogenesis. The proportion of cells with either the normal or the mutation-carrying X chromosome remaining active varies and determines the ability to distinguish carrier state. Carriers with a high proportion of normal X chromosomes remaining active will not show abnormal biochemical test results whereas those with a high proportion of mutation-bearing X chromosomes remaining active are more likely to show biochemical abnormalities. Such individuals may sometimes develop symptoms of the disorder, usually in fairly mild form, and are called manifesting carriers. The problem of lyonisation can be largely overcome if biochemical tests can be performed on clonally derived cells. Hair bulbs have been successfully used to detect carriers of Hunter's syndrome (mucopolysaccharidosis II), by assaying the enzyme iduronate sulphatase.

UK GENETIC TESTING NETWORK (UKGTN)

This is a government-funded body established to co-ordinate molecular genetic testing throughout the UK. It has produced a directory listing all the diseases being tested for in UK laboratories which receive NHS funding. All these tests are scrutinised by the UKGTN Steering Group and a panel of clinicians for their clinical and scientific validity and appropriateness. Some of the diseases listed are very common whereas others have only a handful of cases per year requiring testing. The listing includes inherited metabolic disorders. In the latest version of the directory, 253 diseases are listed.

Molecular genetics services for some important disease (e.g. the prophyrias) are not provided by UKGTN laboratories but are available from other UK service laboratories. A large number of genetic diseases are very rare (one to two families identified each year) and where testing is not available in the UK, samples may be sent to specialist laboratories abroad. Commissioners and regional genetics centres in their area together establish whether provision for these tests is available via NHS funding.

POINTS FOR REFLECTION

- Patients often expect that results will be available within days so it is important to have some idea of how long the results of a particular test may take and to advise the patient at the time of obtaining the sample.
- It is important for families to realise that although a clinical diagnosis may be made, it is not always possible to confirm it with a laboratory test.

REFERENCE

Kallionieni, A. *et al.* (1992) Comparative genomic hybridisation for molecular cytogenetic analysis of solid tumors. *Science*, **258**(5083), 818–21.

5 Risk Perception and Options Available

JO HAYDON

The decisions that individuals make following genetic counselling may depend on how they interpret the information given to them. It is therefore important that information is presented at the appropriate level of understanding for each individual, and this may vary significantly from one person to another, even within the same family. When we talk about risks with a client, we are actually describing the *probability* that an event may occur. Risk figures are often puzzling to individuals who do not have to deal with them on a regular basis. As important decisions will be made on the basis of this understanding, we need to be aware of some of the common factors that can affect individuals' perception of risk.

The way in which risk is determined will also vary. When it is known that a disorder is due to a single gene, a *Mendelian risk* will be given:

- For a dominant disorder this will be 1 in 2 (see Chapter 7).
- For an autosomal recessive disorder or an X-linked recessive disorder, it will be 1 in 4 (see Chapters 8 & 9).

In some situations, when additional information is known about an individual, it may be possible to give a *modified probability*. The process by which the risk is modified is known as a *Bayesian calculation*. Consider the pedigree 5.1.

Individual A (III.1) is asking for her probability of being a carrier for Duchenne muscular dystrophy (DMD). Her maternal grandmother was obviously a carrier as she had two affected sons (the chance of this occurring due to two new mutations would be extremely low).

A's mother therefore had a 1 in 2 probability of being a carrier and A's probability is half of this (1 in 4).

As DMD is inherited as an X-linked condition (see Chapter 9), the risk of a carrier having an affected son is 1 in 4.

A's probability of having a child with Duchenne muscular dystrophy is therefore $1/4 \times 1/4 = 1/16$.

Genetics in Practice: A clinical approach for healthcare practitioners   Edited by Jo Haydon
© 2007 John Wiley & Sons, Ltd

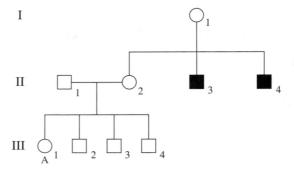

Pedigree 5.1

However, looking at the information contained in the pedigree may help to modify this probability:

- A's mother had three sons, none of whom were affected.
- If A's mother had been a carrier, she would have had a 1 in 2 probability that each son would be affected. As she has three normal sons the modified or 'conditional' probability that she is a carrier is $1/2 \times 1/2 \times 1/2 = 1/8$.
- the probability that she would have three unaffected sons if she was not a carrier is 1.

The joint probability is determined by multiplying the prior probability by the modified/conditional probability:

- The joint probability that she is a carrier is $1/2 \times 1/8 = 1/16$.
- The likelihood that she is not a carrier is $1/2 \times 1 = 1/2 = 8/16$.

The relative probability is a ratio between the risk that she is a carrier and the likelihood that she is not, i.e. 1:8.

The following calculation is now made:

Table 5.1 Bayesian Calculation

Probability	A's mother IS a carrier	A's mother is NOT a carrier
Prior	1/2	1/2
Conditional (3 healthy sons)	$1/2 \times 1/2 \times 1/2 = 1/8$	$1 \times 1 \times 1 = 1$
Joint	$1/2 \times 1/8 = 1/16$	$1/2 \times 1 = 1/2 = 8/16$
Relative risk	1	8
Modified	1/9	8/9

In this situation, if A's mother's probability of being a carrier is calculated to be 1/9:

- A's probability will be half of this, i.e. 1/18.
- A's probability of having a child with Duchenne muscular dystrophy is therefore $1/18 \times 1/4 = 1/72$.

Empiric risk is based on observed data and is the form of risk used for the common non-Mendelian or chromosome disorders. The accuracy of these risks is dependent on data being collected in an unbiased way. It is also important 'that the population from which the individual receiving genetic counselling comes is comparable to the one on which the data were established' (Harper, 2004, p12).

FACTORS AFFECTING RISK PERCEPTION

PRECONCEIVED IDEAS

The preconceived ideas that individuals bring with them to the genetic clinic may affect how well the information given to them is received. Misinformation given previously by family members, professionals or, increasingly commonly, by the media or the internet may be so firmly entrenched in their belief systems that it is difficult for them to accept an altered risk. For example, a male may believe that he is not at risk of developing the dominant condition that his mother had because previously all the affected individuals in his family were females. He may find it difficult to accept that this happened by chance. Similarly, an affected woman with an adult onset dominant condition may believe that her children are not at risk because previously the condition appears to have skipped a generation. This belief may be because her father (whose family had a definite history of the condition) died at an early age, e.g. following a road traffic accident, before the gene mutation that he carried manifested itself. Sometimes these types of misinformation have been given to the family by a medical practitioner who has had limited experience of the condition. Genetic conditions are often featured in soap operas but are usually inaccurately portrayed. There may be misinformation about the symptoms, the mode of inheritance and/or the options available for families with a specific condition. Many newspaper articles have exaggerated the risks associated with familial cancer and used headlines that create anxiety in a large proportion of the population. Many members of the public are surprised to learn that cancer only has a genetic component in about 5–10% of cases. There is also a common belief that a simple gene test is available to all families to determine whether or not an individual is at high risk of developing a specific form of cancer. Some believe that finding a gene mutation for a particular form of cancer means that the individual will definitely develop cancer. Internet sites are not always carefully monitored and clients may arrive at the genetic clinic armed with information from an obscure web site that contains out-of-date or basically wrong information.

UNDERSTANDING THE RISK GIVEN

Risk can be given as odds or as a percentage and the method used may affect the individual's perception of that risk. For example, the risk of a train arriving late at its destination may be presented as 1 in 10 or as 10%:

• Which of these sounds most likely to you and which might cause you concern?

Giving the counterbalance of the chance that an event might *not* occur may also have a significant effect on the way the risk is perceived. Thinking of our train journey, the likelihood of the same train arriving on time may be given as 9 in 10 or 90%:

• Would you be more worried by a 1 in 10 risk of being late or relieved by a 9 in 10 chance or being on time, a 10% risk of being late or a 90% chance of being on time, and which might seem more likely?

Giving the counterbalance of chance also ensures that the individual recognises the difference between the unwanted outcome and a normal outcome occurring. When discussing risks with individuals it is important to try to assess whether odds or a percentage seems more clearly understood. When comparing risk with the counterbalance of chance, it is essential to use the same descriptive terms, e.g. 1/10 or 9/10. To describe the same situation as a 1/10 risk and a 90% chance will cause confusion.

    In some circumstances risk may be presented in relative terms, i.e. high, moderate or low. However, these are objective assessments of the risk. If one is talking about the risk of having a severely affected child with a potentially lethal condition, who is to say whether a 5% risk is high, moderate or low? When describing risks related to breast or bowel cancer, however, it may be relevant to relate the risk to the general population risk for that disorder; thus an individual's risk of developing breast cancer may be described as 'similar to the population risk' (i.e. 10%) rather than as being 11%. Sometimes merely by giving a risk figure, anxiety will be provoked in the client. One might assume that giving someone a 1/400 risk would be reassuring, but the individual may not previously have been aware of any risk being present and may find this worrying, rather than being reassured that there is a 399/400 chance that the event will not occur.

    When discussing risk, whether it is for an individual, other family members or potential offspring, it is important that it is understood that the risk given is for each individual and that it refers to the future not the past, as risk/chance has no memory. For example, if a couple has one affected child and is given a 1/4 (25%) risk of recurrence, it is important that they understand that this risk is for each subsequent child. Some couples might otherwise perceive this as meaning that as they already have one affected child, the next three children will be unaffected.

Another problem in understanding may arise if a couple has had two affected and no unaffected children and is then told there is a 1/4 risk of recurrence. They may perceive their risk as 100% (as to date all of their children are affected) and feel that they have been given incorrect information. Simple ways to explain Mendelian risk to couples may be by comparing it to the toss of a coin. Most people are familiar with the concept that there is an equal chance of the coin landing heads or tails each time the coin is tossed as the coin has no memory and cannot control which side up it will land. A 1/2 risk can therefore be described as 'heads you get it, tails you don't'. A 1/4 risk can be compared to tossing two coins; as long as there is at least one tail showing, the child will be unaffected. There are three possible combinations in which one or both coins land tail-up; the fourth possibility is that both coins land head-up and the child will be affected.

PERSONALITY

An optimist will perceive a risk in a completely different way to a pessimist. Consider a jar of coffee when half the contents have been consumed. An optimist will describe the jar as half full whereas a pessimist will describe it as half empty. The optimist will be reassured by the 9/10 chance that the train will arrive on time whereas the pessimist will be convinced that the 1/10 risk of being late means that they should catch the earlier train to be sure of arriving at their eventual destination on time.

IMPACT (BURDEN) OF THE CONDITION

If a family perceives the care of an affected child to be not much different to that of any normal child then a high risk of 1/2 (50%) may not be viewed as a problem. If, however, the burden of care is perceived as high, then even a low recurrence risk may be regarded as too great to consider having another child.

Two families that were seen within a short time of each other brought these lessons home to the author quite forcibly early in her experience as a genetic counsellor.

Family 1; Mr and Mrs Evans

Mrs Evans' mother, her maternal grandmother and her three great aunts had all been diagnosed with Huntington disease. At that time, the gene for the disorder had not been discovered, so we were only able to tell Mrs Evans that she had a 50% risk of having inherited the gene for this condition and nothing further could be offered to clarify the situation. Much to our surprise, Mrs Evans was delighted with this information as in her family, by chance, all the affected individuals had been females. The myth had therefore developed that in her family females were always affected. By giving her a 50% risk we had also given her a 50% chance of *not* developing the disease and she went away feeling much happier.

Family 2: Mr and Mrs Jones and their two young sons, James aged four and Steven aged two

James looked completely normal but had developmental delay and severe behavioural problems. Taking him out was a nightmare as he frequently threw temper tantrums, screaming and lashing out at his parents. They often heard people commenting that they should have more control over their son and suggesting that he needed a 'good slap'. (How many times might we have passed judgement on an apparently normal but badly behaved child in the supermarket?) He slept for short periods only and not before midnight. A lock had had to be put on the outside of his bedroom door as on a number of occasions James had gone downstairs during the night and smeared faeces over the walls of the dining room. Mr and Mrs Jones felt that their relationship was under severe strain as they rarely had time alone together (James went to bed late and his behaviour prevented the possibility of babysitters). They no longer went out as a family as James's behaviour was so disruptive. They worried about the effect on their younger son, Steven, as they felt he was missing out on normal family experiences. Extensive tests failed to show the reason for James's behaviour and the couple was given an empiric recurrence of risk of 3–5% (with a 95–97% chance that the condition would not recur). Mr Jones summed up his reaction to this risk by saying, 'Even if you told us it was a one in a million that would be too high. We are barely managing to survive in our present situation. If we had another James, we could not possibly cope.' His wife, however, did not regard this risk in the same way. Her relationship with James was closer than her husband's as she was James's main carer. Her strong feelings of love for James lessened her perception of the burden of his care, especially as he was still only four years old and therefore required more attention than an older child would need. Had we seen the couple when James was older, her perception may have been different.

For this couple, therefore, the impact (burden) of the condition was viewed differently, giving them a different perception of the risk of having another child. They were now faced not only with the problem of coping with James and his effect on their lives, but what proved for them to be an in irreconcilable difference of opinion about future reproductive decisions. Mrs Jones was prepared to take the risk but Mr Jones most definitely was not. Sadly, several years later the couple separated.

The perceived burden of the condition may also be affected by the reaction of the extended family to the affected individual. For some families, the extended family is a close-knit unit, with parents still having a lot of influence over decisions made by their adult offspring. In these families, if the affected child is accepted as an equal member, with help being given to the care of the child, the risk of another similarly affected child being born may not be perceived as a major problem. Conversely, if the affected child is seen as defective, or a source of embarrassment, the parents may perceive the child as a greater burden then they would otherwise have done. Sadly, it is not uncommon to hear of grandparents apportioning blame for the condition on their son/daughter-in-law because 'nothing like this has ever happened on our side before'.

TESTS AVAILABLE FOR ADULTS

In the previously mentioned case, Mr and Mrs Jones may both have perceived their risk differently if it had been possible to give a definitive diagnosis and therefore a definite risk. This risk might have been low if the diagnosis had been of a condition known to be sporadic and not genetic. The possibility of treatment for a condition may also influence how the risk is perceived. If a genetic disorder was confirmed but treatment was not available, the possibility of prenatal diagnosis with the option of terminating a pregnancy with an affected foetus might also have influenced their perception of the risk.

Tests available for adults include:

1. Diagnostic
2. Carrier
3. Presymptomatic/Predictive
4. Prenatal.

DIAGNOSTIC

For many conditions, the diagnosis is made on clinical grounds, with a high degree of certainty. Confirmation by the use of a laboratory test often increases the client's confidence in the diagnosis given. In some situations, the clinical picture may not be definitive and therefore a laboratory test will help to confirm or exclude the diagnosis. The test used may be chromosomal, molecular or metabolic (see Chapter 3).

CARRIER

If a condition is inherited in a way that means healthy individuals may be carriers, members of the extended family of an affected individual or a known carrier may wish to determine whether or not they are also carriers. Being a carrier does not affect an individual's general health and is only potentially a problem in relation to reproduction. The potential problem will also vary according to the way in which the condition is inherited.

If a condition is due to a chromosome rearrangement, e.g. a translocation (see Chapter 6), a carrier of the balanced form of the rearrangement may be at risk of reduced fertility, recurrent miscarriages or the live birth of a child with severe physical and/or developmental disabilities.

If a condition is inherited as an autosomal (i.e. not sex-linked) recessive disorder (see Chapter 8), there is only a potential problem if the carrier's partner is also a carrier for that condition, when there will be a 1 in 4 (25%) risk of having an affected child. It may be possible to test the partner to determine their carrier status. For example, with B-thalassaemia it is possible to test individuals without a family history to determine whether or not they are carriers. With cystic fibrosis, however, over 1100 common mutations have been found in the gene and it would not be possible to test for all of these. A partner could be tested for the most common mutations and in their absence his/her risk of being a carrier would be significantly reduced, but not excluded.

If a condition is inherited as an X-linked disorder, there is a possibility that females are carriers for that condition, in which case there will be a 1 in 4 (25%) risk of having an affected son. It may be possible to offer a test to determine their carrier status.

Careful thought should be given before proceeding with carrier testing. The person requesting the test should ask themselves what they would do with the information if they proved to be a carrier. Some individuals have reported feeling stigmatised after discovering that they are a carrier for a certain condition. It may alter the individual's self-image and cause strong feelings of guilt. These guilt feelings can be stronger for those individuals carrying a balanced chromosome rearrangement or an X-linked condition, as they can regard themselves as the sole contributor to the potential problems. It is therefore important to be aware of the possible psychological effects of testing.

PRESYMPTOMATIC/PREDICTIVE

For some individuals who are at risk of an adult-onset disorder, it is possible to offer testing to determine whether or not they carry the gene mutation for that disorder. A positive test can indicate that the individual will definitely become affected ('presymptomatic') or that they are at a high risk of becoming affected ('predictive'). For example, an individual shown to carry the gene mutation for Huntington disease will definitely become affected unless they die young due to some other condition. On the other hand, 20% of women who carry a gene mutation associated with breast cancer will not go on to develop breast cancer.

Finding out whether or not an individual carries a gene mutation has far-reaching effects on their life. The decision to have such a test may depend on whether or not there is any treatment available should the test prove positive. If there is not, the individual needs to consider carefully how they might feel if they get a positive result, as it is not possible to predict the age of onset of a disease. Such knowledge may affect the individual's perception of themselves, their relationships with other family members, partners or potential partners. It can also have significant implications for mortgages, insurance and employment. Having a positive result for one of these tests does not mean that the person has been diagnosed with the condition, but it is often difficult for individuals to accept this. It is usually even more difficult for other family members, employers and even medical personnel to appreciate the difference between prediction and diagnosis. It is therefore normal practice for an individual to be seen on a number of occasions for detailed discussion and counselling before proceeding with such a test.

Box 5.1 Examples of Conditions for which Presymptomatic/Predictive Tests may be Requested

These conditions are inherited in an autosomal dominant fashion, so each individual with an affected parent has a 1 in 2 (50%) risk of inheriting the gene mutation.

1. Familial adenomatous polyposis (FAP)
This is a condition that affects the large bowel, in which thousands of polyps (consisting of adenomatous tissue) develop and, if left *in situ*, will result in bowel cancer. The gene mutation can now be identified in most families and a presymptomatic test is offered to at risk individuals to clarify their situation. Those individuals found to carry the gene mutation can be offered surgery to remove the whole of the large bowel. Although this is a major operation, the success rate is good and the risk of bowel cancer is thus removed.

2. Colon cancer
If an individual is a member of a family known to have a gene mutation in one of the genes that protect against colon cancer, their risk of having inherited such a mutation can be clarified by a predictive test. If they are found to have the mutation, their risk of developing colon cancer is known to be 80% (see Chapter 12) and they can be offered regular colon screening to detect early signs of malignancy should they occur. They can then be offered the appropriate treatment at a much earlier stage than if treatment was only offered when symptoms became apparent.

3. Huntington disease
The offspring of an individual with Huntington disease, which affects movements, personality and cognition, can be offered a presymptomatic test, but in this case there is no preventive treatment available and the age of onset cannot be predicted. All that can be offered following a positive test result is support and counselling.

Uptake of predictive tests
In each of these disorders the risk to offspring of an affected individual is 1 in 2 (50%) but the perception of the severity of the risk may be affected by the subsequent options available. Thus the uptake for predictive testing for FAP, where a treatment can be offered, is far higher than that for HD, where only information can be given.

PRENATAL

Prenatal testing for genetic disorders should not be confused with antenatal screening.

Antenatal Screening Tests

Screening tests are routinely offered to members of a defined population to determine which individuals are at an increased risk of a specific condition. Further tests are then offered to at-risk individuals to determine whether they are affected by the condition. In pregnancy, women are offered screening tests for a number of conditions.

Down Syndrome

A number of different tests may be offered at different stages of pregnancy, looking for either increased or decreased measurements:

1. First trimester (i.e. first 13 weeks of pregnancy).

   • Ultrasound scanning to measure the nuchal translucency (increased). This may also indicate the presence of heart defects.
   • Maternal serum tests to measure pregnancy associated plasma protein-A (PAPP-A) (decreased) and human chorionic gonadotrophin (HCG) (increased).
   • A combination of the nuchal translucence and serum tests.

2. Second trimester (i.e. 14–26 weeks of pregnancy).

   • Double tests for alphafetoprotein (AFP) (decreased) and HCG.
   • Triple test for AFP, HCG and unconjugated estril (uE3) (reduced).
   • Quadruple test for AFP, HCG, uE3 and inhibin A (increased).

3. Integrated testing, which is a combination of:

   • Nuchal translucency measurements in the first trimester.
   • Triple or quadruple maternal serum testing in the second trimester.

Neural tube defects

A high level of AFP may indicate an open neural tube defect or an abdominal wall defect.

Haemoglobinopathy carriers

All women should be offered screening for thalassaemia and sickle cell carrier status. Until recently, these tests were only offered to women from ethnic groups with a higher risk, e.g. African-Caribbean women were offered screening for sickle cell, while Asian women were offered thalassaemia screening. However, it has been recognised that carrier status is not limited to ethnic groups, and with increases in inter-ethnic unions it may be difficult to differentiate between ethnic groups.

All women in high prevalence areas are now offered haemoglobinopathy screening, while women in low prevalence areas are offered testing according to ancestry. If a woman is found to be a carrier, testing should also be offered to her partner. If both partners are found to be carriers, there will be a 1 in 4 (25%) risk to the foetus of whichever condition they are carriers for.

Prior to consenting for any of these tests, the woman should have been given sufficient information to enable her to give informed consent. Despite this, many women still expect the results to bring reassurance and are totally unprepared for an adverse result.

Prenatal Testing for Genetic Disorders

Prenatal testing is now available for a wide range of conditions and has given many couples more freedom to choose whether or not they will embark on further pregnancies. However, the choice is not always an easy one and there are a number of issues that need to be considered. It is important to be aware of the possible reasons for requesting the test, the psychological effects of being tested and the different tests available. These issues will be discussed in a later section.

PREGNANCY OPTIONS

There are three main options available to a couple with a known risk to offspring:

- Avoid further pregnancies.
- Plan further pregnancies

    1. accepting the risk
    2. with prenatal diagnosis
    3. with artificial insemination from a donor
    4. with egg donation
    5. with pre-implantation genetic diagnosis.

- Postpone the decision in the hope that more choices will become available in the near future.

AVOID FURTHER PREGNANCIES

This option may be considered if a couple decides that they do not wish to have an affected child and either no prenatal diagnosis is available or termination of an affected pregnancy would not be acceptable to them. The couple may wish to consider adoption as a possible alternative and it is therefore important to discuss whether or not this might be possible. If an individual is known to carry the gene for Huntington disease, for example, it is unlikely that they would be considered suitable for adoption. The concern would be that the potential parent might become affected with this condition (which usually presents between the ages of 35 and 55 years) before the adopted child had reached adulthood. However, a young woman with Turner syndrome (45, X) who is infertile but expected to have a normal healthy life span should not be excluded from adoption on medical grounds.

PLAN FURTHER PREGNANCIES

Accepting the Risk

If prenatal diagnosis is not available, or if termination of pregnancy would not be acceptable to the couple, they may decide to accept the risk of having an affected child and proceed with a pregnancy regardless of the risk.

With Prenatal Diagnosis

Whatever the reason for requesting the test, it must be remembered that the majority of these pregnancies were planned and, even when unexpected, wanted. The decision to have a prenatal test is not an easy one but the couple may feel that for them it is the only choice they have. The early weeks of a wanted pregnancy are usually associated with great happiness and expectation and the pleasure of telling family and friends the good news. Couples contemplating prenatal diagnosis have the conflicting hopes that the pregnancy will lead to the birth of an unaffected child, worries that the prenatal test may result in miscarriage of a potentially normal baby and fears that a decision about termination may have to be made, together with guilt about contemplating such a choice.

Although it may be possible to arrange prenatal diagnosis when the couple is seen for the first time during a pregnancy, it is preferable for them to have been seen by a member of the genetic team prior to pregnancy occurring. This allows time for discussion and reflection upon the options available, without any pressure to make a hurried decision which may be regretted at a later date.

For some single gene disorders where the gene mutation has not been detected, it may be necessary to compare blood from several family members. This will take time, maybe several months, and cannot therefore be offered if the woman is already pregnant.

Box 5.2 Possible Reasons for Requesting Prenatal Diagnosis

  i) To avoid the birth of an affected child by terminating any pregnancies in which the foetus is found to be affected.

 ii) In rare cases, to know if a foetus is affected so that specific treatment can be carried out while the foetus is *in utero*.

iii) To know in advance and prepare for the treatment that will be required following delivery. This may require the woman to be delivered in a regional

obstetric unit with a neonatal intensive care unit and/or a neonatal surgical unit on site to reduce the need for a very ill baby to be transferred a long distance for treatment.
iv) To relieve uncertainty. For some couples, living with uncertainty throughout the period of pregnancy would be worse than knowing, even if they discover that their baby is affected and they decide to continue with the pregnancy.
The types of tests available will be discussed later in the chapter.

With Artificial Insemination from a Donor (AID)

The couple may opt for artificial insemination of sperm from a donor if the male partner is affected and there is a 1 in 2 (50%) risk, or if both partners are carriers for a recessive condition with a 1 in 4 (25%) risk. Usually when this procedure is carried out as treatment for male sub-fertility, the couple is advised to have intercourse around the time of the insemination so that there is a possibility that conception has occurred spontaneously. When the procedure is being carried out to avoid a genetic disorder, it is most important that the couple does not have unprotected intercourse at this time as the couple's fertility is not in doubt and spontaneous conception could result in an affected child.

With Egg Donation

If the female is affected with a dominant condition or is a carrier for an X-linked condition then the couple may opt for egg donation from another female. This is less easily available and involves *in vitro* fertilisation (IVF). Although the donor is not infertile, she has to be given hormones to stimulate production of eggs, which then have to be removed via the vagina under heavy sedation. If fertilisation is successfully achieved it is normal practice to replace two embryos in the uterus. The chance of achieving a live birth with IVF is around 20%. The risks associated with this process include ovarian hyper-stimulation syndrome for the donor and multiple pregnancy for the couple, not to mention the additional emotional stress involved in achieving a successful pregnancy.

With Pre-Implantation Genetic Diagnosis

This is a relatively new procedure that is only available in a limited number of centres. Although the couple does not usually have a fertility problem, the process requires *in vitro* fertilisation. About 2–3 days after fertilisation has occurred, when the blastocyst is at the 8-cell stage, one cell is removed and analysed for the specific disorder involved. Only embryos shown to be unaffected by the genetic disorder under investigation will be returned to the uterus (maximum of two embryos). The chance of achieving a live birth is the same as for any *in vitro* fertilisation, i.e. around 20%, and carries the same risks as described in the section on egg donation. As only one cell can be examined, the number of disorders for which the test can be offered is limited. There is also a slight possibility of misdiagnosis (the risk depending on the particular test being carried out) as the results cannot be checked on a second cell, and for this reason couples are advised that the procedure reduces the risk rather than eliminating it and that prenatal diagnosis is recommended. As most couples have chosen this procedure to avoid the need for prenatal diagnosis and possible termination of pregnancy, this may not be acceptable to them. It is important for the couple to realise that only one test can be carried out. For example, if a woman aged 39 years requests the test because she and her partner are carriers for cystic fibrosis and have a 1 in 4 risk of having an affected child, the cell cannot also be tested to exclude Down syndrome.

Centres offering this service to clients usually offer an initial appointment as soon as possible (often within three months) after receiving the referral so that the couple is made aware of all the implications of the process. This means that any couple that decides not to proceed with the process will not have been made to wait a long time before having to rethink their plans for the future. Once a couple decides to proceed with the process, there will be a period of waiting while a license is obtained from the Human Fertility and Embryology Authority and the laboratory performs the necessary technical workup.

POSTPONE THE DECISION

A young couple may decide to postpone plans for pregnancy for a few years in the hope that prenatal testing will become available. This option depends on the age of the woman and the likelihood that a test will become available in the near future.

TYPES OF TEST AVAILABLE IN PREGNANCY

Chorionic Villus Sampling (CVS)

This test is offered at 11–12 weeks of pregnancy. If it is carried out earlier than this there is a risk of foetal damage and an increased risk of miscarriage. A dating scan is therefore recommended at 9 weeks to confirm the dates. During the procedure, a few cells are taken from the developing placenta (afterbirth) and these cells are suitable for chromosome, DNA and biochemical tests.

The test takes place in the ultrasound department and is performed by an experienced obstetrician. It is not available at all obstetric units and the patient may therefore have to attend a different unit to the one in which the remainder of her pregnancy care will be given. An ultrasound scan will check the gestation of the foetus and locate the position of the placenta, and the patient will need a full bladder to facilitate this. The test can be carried out abdominally or vaginally, under ultrasound guidance. A fragment of placental tissue is removed using gentle suction.

The risk of miscarriage following CVS is variable from centre to centre and ranges between 1 in 20 and 1 in 100 (1–5%). The results of the test will normally be available within 3–10 days. If an abnormal result is obtained and the couple decides to terminate the pregnancy, the method used will depend on the gestation period.

The Royal College of Obstetricians and Gynaecologists recommends that suction termination is only carried out up to 12 weeks' gestation. In some cases the result of the test will be available within this time limit. If the pregnancy is further advanced before the result is available, termination will be by medical induction.

CVS gives the woman the chance to have a prenatal test before the pregnancy is obvious to others. The couple may decide not to tell family and friends unless the results are normal and the pregnancy continues, in which case they will be coping with their anxieties without the help and support of important others in their lives. Clients often say the days between having the test and receiving the results seem like the longest in their lives; it can be an agonising time. When professionals offer support it is important that it is given to both members of the couple, as it is easy for the male partner to feel that his needs and concerns are being ignored.

Amniocentesis

This test is usually carried out at about 16 weeks, although in some centres it is offered a little earlier at 14 weeks. A small amount of the amniotic fluid, which surrounds the foetus in the uterus, is removed. The fluid contains skin and bladder cells that have been shed by the foetus. If a gene test is required, foetal cells have to be grown in the laboratory before sufficient DNA can be obtained. The results will therefore take longer than with CVS.

The test takes place in the ultrasound department and is performed by an obstetrician. Under the guidance of ultrasound, a fine needle is passed through the abdominal skin into the uterus. A small amount of amniotic fluid (10–20 mls) is withdrawn into a syringe. The risk of miscarriage following amniocentesis is between 1 in 100 and 1 in 150 (0.75–1%).

In the laboratory, the foetal cells are removed from the amniotic fluid and placed in a culture medium to encourage growth (see Chapter 3). Chromosomes can only be visualised through a microscope during meiosis and therefore the foetal cells have to be encouraged to grow. The results of the test normally take 2–3 weeks. If an abnormal result is obtained and the patient opts to terminate the pregnancy, this will have to be carried out by inducing labour and delivering the foetus vaginally. Otherwise damage may be done to the cervix, which could lead to cervical weakness and late miscarriage in future pregnancies.

In some laboratories a rapid result can be obtained by use of a technique called QF-PCR (see Chapter 3). This is used to determine the sex of the foetus and whether or not trisomies 21, 18 & 13 are present. This test may not always be available on the NHS.

Foetal Blood Sampling (FBS)

This test is only carried out in a few specialist foetal medicine departments. It is usually performed at 18–22 weeks of pregnancy. A small sample of foetal blood is taken from the umbilical cord or a small blood vessel in the foetal abdomen. This sample is suitable for chromosome, DNA and biochemical tests.

The test is performed by an experienced consultant in foetal medicine. The procedure is carried out under ultrasound guidance. A fine needle is passed into the uterus and into the umbilical cord of the foetus. When the needle is in position, a small sample of blood is withdrawn into a syringe. The risk of miscarriage following FBS for genetic testing is around 1 in 100 (1%). The risk of miscarriage is higher when the test is carried out for non-genetic reasons, e.g. rhesus incompatibility, when the foetal condition is already likely to be compromised.

If an abnormal result is obtained and the patient opts to terminate the pregnancy, this will have to be carried out by inducing labour and delivering the foetus vaginally.

Chorionic villus sampling, amniocentesis and foetal blood sampling all carry a risk of miscarriage due to their invasive nature. A client may go home after any of these procedures, but is advised to rest for the remainder of the day and to avoid strenuous exercise for the next few days. Arrangements should be made for giving the results. This is usually done via the telephone and it is common practice to arrange to contact a client at a time when her partner is likely to be with her. It is also advisable to discuss with the couple what they will do if the test shows that the foetus is affected. If the couple is sure that their decision will be to terminate the pregnancy, they may wish the obstetrician to be informed of the results before them so that arrangements for an appointment can be made. The genetic counsellor can then inform the couple of these arrangements at the same time as giving the results. When giving bad news, clients usually appreciate a direct but sympathetic approach. However hard it is for the genetic counsellor to give the bad news, it cannot compare to the distress that the couple will feel when receiving it.

Ultrasound Scanning (USS)

This is a safe, non-invasive test in which sound waves are passed through the abdomen and reflected back from the various tissues in the uterus to give an image of the uterine contents. It can be routinely used to assess the gestation of the foetus in early pregnancy and to look for obvious structural abnormalities at around 20 weeks' gestation.

When there is a specific risk of the foetus being affected with a genetic condition involving structural abnormalities, detailed scans may be carried out by a senior radiographer or foetal medicine consultant at various stages throughout the pregnancy. These detailed scans cannot usually be carried out until at least 18 weeks' gestation and it may be later still before the condition can be definitely confirmed or excluded. It is therefore important for the couple to consider what action they will take if an abnormality is detected later in the pregnancy, i.e. after 20 weeks.

If an abnormal result is obtained and the patient opts to terminate the pregnancy, this will have to be carried out by inducing labour and delivering the foetus vaginally.

Support will be needed for those couples whose pregnancies are affected, whatever their decision. If they continue with the pregnancy they may experience feelings of loss and bereavement for the normal baby that they had hoped to have, even as they are trying to look forward to the birth of the child they have chosen. If they terminate the pregnancy they may experience profound feelings of loss and bereavement, anger that they are in such a situation and a sense of guilt that they chose to end the pregnancy. The experience of termination, however sensitively handled by professionals, can be traumatic. Additional stress may be caused by the desire to keep the reason for their admission secret from other patients on the ward. The couple may also feel that the pregnancy, and the accompanying hopes and expectations, physical discomforts and anxieties about the test, has been a waste of time, as they are left with nothing. Undergoing termination may also increase the couple's fears and anxieties when contemplating a future pregnancy.

CASE STUDY: MR AND MRS EVANS' EXPERIENCE OF PRENATAL DIAGNOSIS AND TERMINATION OF PREGNANCY

Mr and Mrs Evans had a son with an unbalanced translocation, leading to both physical problems and severe learning difficulties. Mrs Evans was found to be a carrier for the balanced form of the translocation. When Mrs Evans became pregnant again, the couple opted for prenatal testing, which showed that the baby would have the same unbalanced form as their son. The couple decided they had no option but to terminate the pregnancy as they felt unable to give two affected children the amount of care and stimulus they needed. However, the couple found the experience of terminating the pregnancy very painful and took many months to recover. They felt very guilty that they had taken the decision to end a potential child's life. They also felt very angry that this had happened to them, and that all their pre-conceptual care with diet and avoidance of alcohol and smoking had been in vain.

Several years later they felt emotionally ready to embark on a further pregnancy. When Mrs Evans had her dating scan, a missed abortion was diagnosed. Although very distressed by the loss of another pregnancy, Mr and Mrs Evans both found it easier to grieve as they felt no guilt about the loss. In a subsequent pregnancy, prenatal diagnosis showed that the baby had normal chromosomes. The couple was able to enjoy the remainder of that pregnancy.

TESTING CHILDREN

The general consensus within the genetics community is that genetic tests should only performed on children if there is a diagnostic/clinical indication.

Predictive/presymptomatic testing should only be carried out at the request of the individual to be tested. If parents were to make the decision to have a child tested they would be denying the child the right to make their own choice when they are old enough to understand the implications. Not only would the child be denied that right, but if a positive result were obtained it might influence the way the parents interacted with the child (e.g. being unnecessarily over-protective, limiting their activities) and have profound effects on the child's choices in relation to occupation, life insurance and mortgages.

One obvious exception to the rule against presymptomatic testing is in the case of familial adenomatous polyposis (FAP) (see Box 5.1). In this condition, it is known that the polyps may start appearing from early teen years. Before DNA tests were available, children at risk of developing the condition were offered annual colonoscopies from the age of 11–12 years. This is an uncomfortable and embarrassing procedure for young teenagers (not without risk of damage to the bowel) and many failed to comply with the suggested testing. For many families a DNA test to determine whether or not the mutation is present is now available, and this has led to a great reduction in the number of individuals needing colonoscopy. Also, there is a greater likelihood of compliance if an individual knows they will be affected rather than that they might be. It is recommended that children at risk of developing FAP are seen when they are about 11–12 years old to discuss the tests available and the options open to them if they carry the gene mutation.

For other adult-onset disorders, presymptomatic/predictive testing is not offered until the child has reached the age of 16 years. Occasionally there are exceptional circumstances when a child requests the test at an earlier age. These would have to be considered on an individual basis.

In the case of carrier testing for a balanced translocation, an autosomal recessive disorder or an X-linked condition, it is recommended that the issue is discussed with the child when they are around 16 years of age. They are then able to decide for themselves if they wish to be tested.

POINTS FOR REFLECTION

- The concept of risk may be a difficult one for families to grasp – as you may be aware if you struggled at the beginning of this chapter!

- What strategies might you employ when helping individuals to consider the choices available to them?
- How easy would you find it to support a couple making decisions about a pregnancy that you might find personally unacceptable?
- Are you aware of the non-verbal messages that you may be giving to individuals?

REFERENCE

Harper, P.S. (2004) *Practical Genetic Counselling*, 6th edn, Arnold, London.

6 Chromosome Disorders

JO HAYDON

Chapter 2 looked at chromosomes in detail and reminded us that the discovery that a normal human cell contains 46 chromosomes was made as recently as 1956. The chromosomes are arranged in 23 pairs. The first 22 pairs, known as autosomes, are numbered 1 to 22 by size (number 1 being the largest). The 23rd pair determines the sex of the individual, females having two X chromosomes and males having one X and one Y chromosome. The exceptions to this rule are the gametes, the eggs and the sperm. During their development, at meiosis, the chromosome pairs separate and one from each pair passes into the egg or the sperm. Thus the egg contains 23 chromosomes, one of each autosome and one X. The sperm also contains 23 chromosomes, one of each autosome and either one X or one Y chromosome. Thus it is the male partner who determines the sex of the foetus. At conception, the new cell that will develop into a foetus contains the full set of 46 chromosomes.

The chromosomes within a cell can be clearly seen through a microscope during the metaphase of cell division (see Chapter 3). The picture thus obtained is known as the karyotype and its description contains information about the number of chromosomes per cell, the composition of the sex chromosomes and any chromosome abnormalities that may be present.

A normal female karyotype would be described as 46, XX, while a normal male karyotype would be described as 46, XY.

Each chromosome is divided into two parts, or arms, by the centromere (see Chapter 3). The short arm of the chromosome is referred to by the letter p and the long arm by the letter q. The tips of both the p and the q arms are known as the telomeres.

Genetics in Practice: A clinical approach for healthcare practitioners   Edited by Jo Haydon
© 2007 John Wiley & Sons, Ltd

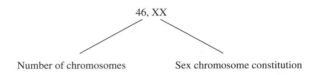

Figure 6.1 A Normal Female Karyotype.

Chromosome abnormalities can be divided into those characterised by differences in number and those characterised by differences in structure. Abnormalities may give rise to recognised patterns known as syndromes.

WHAT IS A SYNDROME?

A syndrome is a combination of signs and symptoms that fit a recognisable pattern. Thus, Down syndrome is frequently recognised by members of the public because of the generalised appearance (known as the gestalt), even if they can't describe its individual features. Whenever a congenital abnormality is noted following birth or later in childhood, it is important that the baby is given a careful physical examination to detect any other problems that may be associated with a syndromic condition. For example, a cleft palate may occur as an isolated condition requiring corrective surgery. If micrognathia (a receding chin) is also noted, the two signs together indicate Pierre Robin syndrome, which requires careful nursing prior to surgery to prevent the tongue being swallowed. Nasogastric tube feeding may also be required prior to surgery.

Once the diagnosis of a syndrome is made, more information about the condition and the possible prognosis will be available. When parents are given the name of a syndrome they may be devastated, as this confirms that there is definitely something wrong with their child. On the other hand, they may be relieved that a diagnosis has been made as this means the condition is not an unknown quality, that there is more information about it available to them, and that there is perhaps a support group that they can contact.

NUMERICAL CHROMOSOME ABNORMALITIES

When an individual whole chromosome is in excess or missing, this is known as aneuploidy. It can happen to either the autosomal chromosomes (1–22) or the sex chromosomes (X and Y) and occurs when there is an error at meiosis. Normally at this stage in cell division one copy of each chromosome passes into each of the two daughter cells. If non-disjunction occurs (see Chapter 2), both copies of the chromosome will be passed into one daughter cell and no copies into the second daughter cell. Fertilisation of these cells will result in a conceptus with either three copies of a chromosome (trisomy) or only one copy (monosomy) in each cell.

AUTOSOMAL ANEUPLOIDIES

Trisomy of any of the autosomal chromosomes may occur at conception but most will result in early miscarriage. Monosomy of an autosomal chromosome is not compatible with life.

Autosomal trisomy is associated with increased maternal age. In females, meiosis in the egg cells begins during uterine life. At birth, ovaries contain hundreds of immature egg cells. Following puberty, each month several of these cells complete meiosis and mature in preparation for ovulation. The older a woman is at conception, the longer these egg cells have been subjected to possible adverse environmental factors before maturing into an ovum.

Trisomy 21: Down Syndrome (47, XX, +21 or 47, XY, +21)

This is the most commonly recognised chromosome abnormality.

Features include hypertelorism (wide spaced eyes), down-slanted eyes, protuberant tongue, round shaped skull, incurved little fingers, single palmar crease and marked muscle hypotonia as a baby. Around 40% of children with Down syndrome will also have congenital heart abnormalities, which can range from mild to severe. As well as the obvious physical features, there will be delayed development, again ranging from mild to severe. Individuals with Down syndrome may live well into adult life but face the added possibility of developing leukaemia and/or early dementia.

Trisomy 18: Edward's Syndrome (47, XX, +18 or 47, XY, +18)

Features include low birth weight, low-set and malformed ears, clenched hands with overlapping fingers, feet with unusual shape due to convex soles (known as 'rocker bottom' feet) and prominent heels. Most babies with this condition will have a congenital heart defect such as ventricular septal defect or a patent ductus arteriosus, and kidney defects may also be present. As well as the physical features, there is severe developmental delay. Ninety percent of infants with trisomy 18 die within the first six months of life.

Trisomy 13: Patau's Syndrome (47, XX, +13 or 47, XY, +13)

Features include low birth weight, microcephaly, cleft lip and/or palate, extra digits (polydactyly) on hands and/or feet and heart and renal defects. As well as the physical features there is severe developmental delay. Ninety seven percent of infants with trisomy 13 die within the first six months of life.

SEX CHROMOSOME ANEUPLOIDIES

XXY: Klinefelter Syndrome (47, XXY)

Approximately 1 in 500–1000 males is born with an extra X chromosome, resulting in the condition known as Klinefelter syndrome. This is probably the most common chromosomal variation found in humans. The syndrome is characterised by tall stature, small testes, scant body hair and infertility. Breast development may appear after puberty. In some cases intellectual difficulty may be experienced, most commonly in verbal skills. Adolescent boys may experience psychological problems with self-image and tend to be shy. There is a wide range of expression of the condition and many men are only diagnosed when they are investigated for infertility, having experienced no problems prior to this.

XYY Syndrome (47, XYY)

Approximately 1 in 1000 males is born with an extra Y chromosome. Most of them will never know they have this condition as they have no reason to have their chromosomes checked. Boys with XYY syndrome may have some delay in speech and may need some extra help at school, but the majority of these boys manage well at mainstream school. A report by Jacobs *et al.* in 1965 suggested that a significant proportion of men detained in a maximum security hospital had an XYY karyotype. However, subsequent studies looking at men in the general population showed a similar incidence of men with an XYY karyotype (Buchanan, 1997). Unfortunately, some professionals are unaware of the later studies and still associate this karyotype with an increased incidence of violence. This can lead to couples making a decision about whether or not to continue their pregnancy based on inaccurate information.

Triple X Syndrome (47, XXX)

Approximately 1 in 1000 females is born with an additional X chromosome. Most of them will never know they have this condition as they have no reason to have their chromosomes checked. Girls with triple X syndrome may be a little later with walking and starting to use single words. They may attend mainstream school but will benefit from additional help.

Monosomy X: Turner Syndrome (45, X)

Approximately 1 in 2500 girls is born with a lack of the second X chromosome, resulting in the condition known as Turner syndrome. The main features of the syndrome are short stature and infertility. The growth rate may be normal for the first two or three years, before slowing down. Although girls with Turner syndrome do not have growth hormone deficiency, growth hormone is often used to increase adult height. In girls with Turner syndrome, the ova degenerate and disappear in early childhood and the ovaries stop working well before the age of puberty. Puberty will usually only occur if replacement oestrogen therapy is given. Girls with Turner syndrome have a normal uterus and vagina and will be able to have an entirely normal sex life, but in 99% of cases will be infertile. However, successful pregnancies have been achieved in some women by assisted conception using donor eggs and *in vitro* fertilisation.

Intelligence in girls with Turner syndrome is usually normal, although there may be some difficulties in spatial awareness and maths, which will benefit from extra help.

Each of the sex chromosome aneuploidies described above has a very low recurrence rate.

CASE STUDY 1: UNEXPECTED DIAGNOSIS AFTER DELIVERY

Jenny, aged 25 years, was well throughout her first pregnancy and all screening tests and ultrasound scans had appeared normal. She and her husband Tony were eagerly awaiting the birth of their first child. However, during labour foetal distress occurred and the baby was delivered with the aid of forceps. The baby, a girl, was in poor condition at birth, with low Apgar scores and abnormal heart sounds. She also had low-set, malformed ears, clenched hands and 'rocker bottom' feet. An ultrasound scan showed a severe ventricular septal defect which would require urgent surgery if the baby was to survive. The baby was transferred to the neonatal unit and the paediatrician requested an urgent consultation with a geneticist. The geneticist agreed with the paediatrician's suspicions that the baby had a chromosome abnormality, most likely trisomy 18, and blood was taken for urgent chromosome analysis.

The geneticist discussed the suspicions with the parents. It was obvious that the little girl would not survive without cardiac surgery, but, if she had trisomy 18, even with successful surgery her prognosis was poor. By the time the blood result confirming the diagnosis of trisomy 18 was available, the parents had decided that if it were diagnosed, they would not subject their daughter to the trauma of surgery when it could not correct her underlying condition. They felt that they wanted to spare her that additional pain and the resultant need for her to be nursed in an intensive care unit with intravenous infusions and monitors attached. They wanted to be able to remain with her and nurse her for the remainder of her short life. The baby, named Helen, was transferred to the parents' room of the neonatal unit and died peacefully in her mother's arms 20 hours later.

A month later, as previously agreed, the genetic counsellor visited the family at their home to provide counselling following the recent bereavement and to answer any questions the couple might have about the risk of recurrence. Jenny and Tony were naturally very sad, but were glad that the diagnosis had been made quickly so that they could spare Helen the pain of surgery and enable her to spend time with them in the privacy of the parents' room.

Jenny and Tony hoped to have more children in the future, once they had allowed themselves time to grieve for the loss of Helen. They would always be sad at losing her and did not want to rush into another pregnancy to try to replace her. They were relieved to hear that, as the blood test had shown that the trisomy occurred due to non-disjunction at meiosis, the risk of a similar chromosome problem in a future pregnancy was low, around 1%.

They asked if prenatal diagnosis would be available in a future pregnancy for added reassurance and were pleased to hear that chorionic villus sampling or amniocentesis would be available if they wished. At that stage they did not feel that they needed to see the counsellor again but knew that they could request a further appointment at any time.

CASE STUDY 2: PRENATAL TEST TO EXCLUDE DOWN SYNDROME: UNEXPECTED RESULTS

During her third pregnancy, Mrs Graham, aged 37, opted for an amniocentesis to exclude the possibility of Down syndrome. The results of the test showed that the baby did not have Down syndrome but was a male with an extra X chromosome (47, XXY), causing Klinefelter syndrome. Mrs Graham and her husband were naturally distressed when given this information as they had hoped that the test result would be normal. Added to this was their uncertainty about what the condition involved. They knew what Down syndrome was and had already decided that they would terminate the pregnancy if that condition was diagnosed. But they had never heard of Klinefelter syndrome and had no idea how serious it might be. The fact that it involved a sex chromosome added to their concerns. The couple was referred to the clinical genetics unit and an urgent appointment was made so that they could find out more about the condition before deciding what action to take.

The geneticist spent some time with the couple, discussing the possible effects of the additional chromosome on the baby (as detailed above). The couple had many questions, including whether or not this would interfere with the boy's sexual ability or would increase his likelihood of being homosexual. The geneticist explained that although the child would be infertile, his sexual function and his sexual orientation would not be affected. The couple also wanted to know the risk of recurrence and was reassured that this was unlikely to happen again.

Mr and Mrs Graham decided to continue with the pregnancy. They were then asked if they would like to be put in touch with a family that had a boy with Klinefelter syndrome. They were pleased to be given this option but felt that they would prefer to wait until after the delivery. It is not usual practice to offer this contact before a couple has made the decision as to whether or not to continue with the pregnancy as to do so may be regarded as implying that they should not terminate the pregnancy.

CASE STUDY 3: TURNER SYNDROME DIAGNOSED DURING INVESTIGATION OF INFERTILITY

Sarah had always been regarded as 'petite' by her family and friends but was quite happy with her height. She was not so happy when breast development and the appearance of axillary and pubic hair occurred much later than in her friends and at a much slower rate. She also became concerned when she had not begun to menstruate by the age of 16. Eventually Sarah and her mother saw their GP, who referred Sarah to a paediatrician. The paediatrician suspected that Sarah might have Turner syndrome and discussed this possibility before taking blood for chromosome analysis. The results of the test confirmed the diagnosis and the paediatrician suggested referral for genetic counselling.

The genetic counsellor saw Sarah with her mother and described the features of Turner syndrome in detail. Sarah was anxious to know if she would be able to have normal sexual relationships and was reassured to hear that she would. She was most upset at the fact that she would be infertile. It was important for the counsellor to discuss the various options that might be available to Sarah if she wished to have children. One possible option was for her to have assisted conception using donor eggs and *in vitro* fertilisation. Another option that she might want to consider would be adoption. The fact that Sarah had Turner syndrome had no implications for her general health and would not, therefore, be a contraindication to adoption.

The counsellor gave Sarah and her mother information about the Turner Syndrome Support Society and suggested that they might like to make contact. The support group holds annual national meetings in the UK, which include sessions for young adolescents with this syndrome to get together and share their worries and concerns, as well as their achievements. Sarah seemed keen to contact the group and was pleased to hear that there were other girls of a similar age with her condition that she might be able to meet. She described 'feeling like a freak' when she was first told about her chromosome abnormality and was relieved to hear that it was a well recognised disorder and not as rare as she had first assumed.

Following the consultation, the counsellor wrote to Sarah summarising their discussion, and a copy of the letter was sent to her GP and paediatrician. This is normal practice in clinical genetics and helps to reinforce the information given during the consultation. Sarah could also choose to show the letter to relatives or friends so that she could explain the condition more easily.

STRUCTURAL CHROMOSOME ABNORMALITIES

It is known that chromosomes may break and then rejoin (see Chapter 2). Structural abnormalities occur when there are breaks in chromosomes that lead to a net loss, gain or abnormal rearrangement of one or more chromosomes. As laboratory techniques have improved, smaller and subtler structural abnormalities have been detected which would previously have gone unnoticed.

RECIPROCAL TRANSLOCATIONS

Balanced reciprocal translocations occur when two non-homologous (different) chromosomes break and the resulting detached segments swap places with each other. For example, a chromosome 1 and a chromosome 5 may both break while lying adjacent to each other. One piece of chromosome 1 may join to a piece of chromosome 5 and the second piece of chromosome 1 join to a second piece of chromosome 5. There is, therefore, exchange of chromosomal material between the two chromosomes, but no chromosomal material is lost or gained, just rearranged (see Figure 6.2).

About 1 in 500 people carry a balanced reciprocal translocation. They are known as balanced translocation carriers and are clinically normal. The translocation will have no effect on their health. However, carriers of a balanced translocation can have problems when they reproduce. It is possible for a balanced translocation carrier to pass on the translocation in an unbalanced form. This results in a foetus with too much of one chromosome and not enough of another (see Figure 6.4), which may result in spontaneous miscarriage or the birth of a live baby with physical and/or developmental problems. Male translocation carriers may also have reduced fertility.

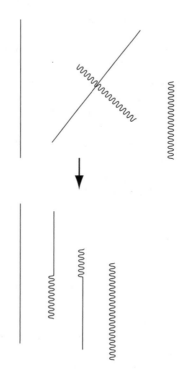

Figure 6.2 Breakage and Realignment of Chromosomes to Form a Reciprocal Translocation.

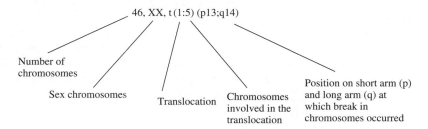

Figure 6.3 Karyotype of a Female with a Balanced Translocation between the Long Arm of Chromosome 1 and the Short Arm of Chromosome 5.

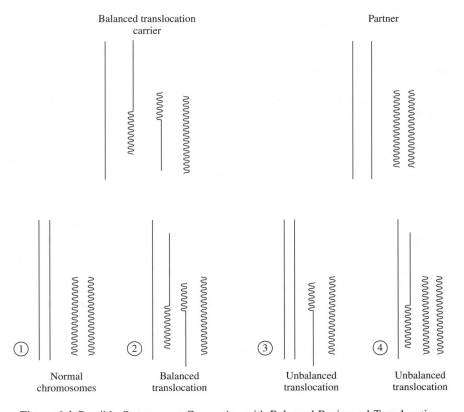

Figure 6.4 Possible Outcomes at Conception with Balanced Reciprocal Translocation.

In some families with balanced reciprocal translocations there is a history of multiple miscarriages but no live-born affected babies. In these families it may be that both forms of the unbalanced chromosomes lead to miscarriage. In this situation a couple may decide not to have an invasive prenatal test but to request a detailed ultrasound scan to exclude major abnormalities. A normal scan may give reassurance but there will always be a small residual risk of a live-born child with an unbalanced translocation leading to physical and/or developmental problems. In some cases the laboratory is able to quantify this risk.

CASE STUDY 4: RECIPROCAL TRANSLOCATION DIAGNOSED AFTER INFANT DEATH

Claire and Roger were referred for genetic counselling several months after their two month old son, Jordan, died from multiple abnormalities. Before he died, Jordan's chromosomes had been checked and it was found that he had an abnormal chromosome 4. Blood had been taken from both Claire and Roger to try to determine the source of this extra material. Roger's chromosomes were normal but Claire was found to have a balanced translocation between chromosome 4 and 11. Claire was devastated by this news and felt very guilty that she had caused Jordan's problems. This result also explained Claire's previous miscarriage. The couple had no living children and felt that they would never be able to have a normal healthy child. They were seeing a bereavement counsellor at the hospital where Jordan had been treated and were slowly coming to terms with their loss. When Claire and Roger felt ready to find out more about the translocation, they were referred for genetic counselling.

The genetic counsellor spent some time with the couple, discussing their feelings about the loss of their son. A detailed family history was then obtained. This revealed that Claire's mother, Mary, had also had several miscarriages and a daughter, Catherine, who had died when a few weeks old with multiple problems similar to Jordan's. Claire's brother Michael and his wife were awaiting an appointment for investigations of infertility as they had been trying to conceive for two years without success. Claire's maternal grandmother had also had several miscarriages and a daughter who died in infancy with congenital abnormalities. There was no history of note in Roger's family.

There were a number of issues that the genetic counsellor needed to discuss with this couple:

1. possible outcomes in future pregnancies
2. options available in future pregnancies
3. implications for the extended family.

The GC was able to reassure Claire and Roger that despite their experiences so far, they had a good chance of having normal, healthy children in the future. With the aid of diagrams, she explained the possible outcomes in future pregnancies

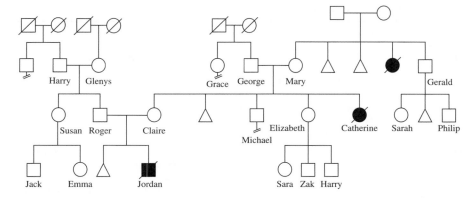

Pedigree 6.1

(see Figure 6.4). Despite their understanding of the information given, the couple still found it hard to accept this, due to their previous experience. The GC showed them the family pedigree that she had drawn and explained how this suggested that Claire's mother, Mary, was also likely to be a carrier. Although Mary had had two miscarriages and an affected daughter, she had also had three healthy children, which proved that this was possible with this particular translocation. This gave Claire and Roger some hope, but they were keen to know if there were tests available in pregnancy that would examine the baby's chromosomes. They knew that early pregnancy would always be an anxious time for them and felt that they would not be able to cope with another pregnancy unless they knew that the baby had normal (or balanced) chromosomes. The GC explained that there would be two prenatal tests available to them to determine this information:

1. chorionic villus sampling (CVS), carried out at 11 weeks' gestation, results available within 7–10 days, miscarriage rate of 1–2% in her local unit.
2. amniocentesis, carried out at 16 weeks' gestation, results available within 2–3 weeks; miscarriage rate of 0.5–1% (see Chapter 5 for more details about prenatal tests).

Claire and Roger then discussed the advantages and disadvantages of these tests with the genetic counsellor (see Table 6.1).

Some couples in this situation opt for CVS as there is a definite possibility of a live-born child with severe problems, while others opt for amniocentesis so that if the pregnancy is going to miscarry, this will already have happened spontaneously. Claire and Roger did not have to make a decision about prenatal testing at this point but it was important for them to be aware of what would be available in a future pregnancy.

Having clarified the situation for themselves, the couple was anxious to know of any possible implications for other family members. The GC suggested that they

Table 6.1 Advantages and Disadvantages of Prenatal Tests Available

	CVS	AMNIOCENTESIS
Advantages	Result within first trimester (13 weeks) of pregnancy Pregancy not yet obvious to other people. Termination of pregnancy *may* be available under general anaesthetic	Lower miscarriage rate
Disadvantages	Higher miscarriage rate	Results not available until 18–19 weeks' gestation Pregnancy may be obvious to others Termination always involves induced labour

approach Claire's parents and offer them the opportunity to be tested. Although it looked likely that Claire's mother was a translocation carrier, the test would be offered to both parents, partly for accuracy and partly to reduce any feelings of guilt that might be induced in Mary. Claire felt that her mother would be anxious to clarify the situation as she had already referred to the fact that there seemed to be 'something' in her side of the family that was causing problems. If Mary was found to be a carrier then Michael and Elizabeth could also be offered testing, as well as Gerald, Mary's only remaining sibling. Although he and his wife would not be having more children, if he was found to be a translocation carrier the test could be offered to his two existing children. If Mary's husband George was found to be a carrier, his sister could be offered testing, but might not want it as she had no offspring. Offering tests to the extended family in this way is known as cascade testing (see Chapter 5).

Claire and Roger were going to continue with bereavement counselling so did not feel that they would need to see the GC again at this point. They would talk to Claire's parents about the blood test and let the GC know the outcome. If Claire's parents declined testing (which Claire felt was unlikely) then the test could be offered to Claire's sister and brothers.

The couple also said that they would contact the GC as soon as another pregnancy occurred, as they felt that they would need her support during a future pregnancy, whatever decisions they made about testing.

ROBERTSONIAN TRANSLOCATIONS

Robertsonian translocations can only occur between two acrocentric chromosomes, which are those chromosomes with centromeres close to the top end (numbers 13, 14, 15, 21 and 22). This form of translocation occurs when two acrocentric chromosomes break at or close to their centromeres. The two short arms are lost and the long arms fuse to form one chromosome (the loss of the short arms of these chromosomes is known to be of no clinical significance as they contain no essential genetic material). The total number of chromosomes is thus reduced to 45.

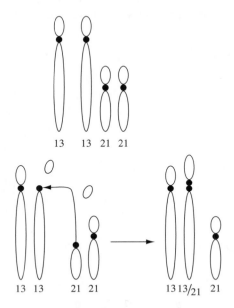

Figure 6.5 Diagram Showing Breakage and Realignment of Chromosomes to Form a Robertsonian Translocation.

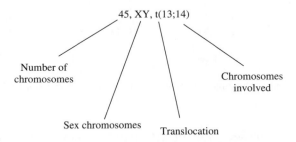

Figure 6.6 Karyotype of a Male with a Balanced Robertsonian Translocation between Chromosomes 13 and 14.

About 1 in 1000 people carries a balanced Robertsonian translocation. They are clinically normal and it will have no effect on their health. However, carriers of a balanced Robertsonian translocation can have problems when they reproduce. It is possible for a balanced translocation carrier to pass on the translocation in an unbalanced form. This results in a foetus with either a missing or an extra long arm of a chromosome (see Figure 6.7), which may result in spontaneous miscarriage or the birth of a live baby with physical and/or developmental problems. Male Robertsonian translocation carriers may also have reduced fertility.

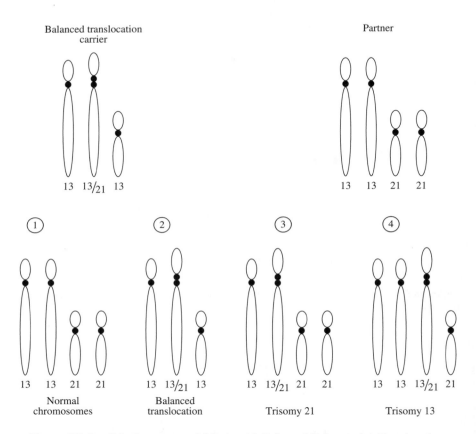

Figure 6.7 Possible Outcomes at Meiosis with Balanced Robertsonian Translocation.

CASE STUDY 5: DOWN SYNDROME DUE TO ROBERTSONIAN TRANSLOCATION

When Kate booked in her first pregnancy, a brief family history was taken. Kate was an only child whose parents had been killed in a road traffic accident shortly after her marriage. Her partner, Martin, was one of four siblings. His mother, Mary, thought that her youngest sibling, a boy who had died shortly after birth due to a congenital heart abnormality, might have had Down syndrome. Mary's mother (Martin's grandmother) had been 45 years old at the time and the cause of Down syndrome had been attributed to advanced maternal age. Kate's first pregnancy resulted in the birth of a healthy son, James. Sadly, each of Kate's next three pregnancies ended in first trimester miscarriage. The obstetrician therefore arranged for blood to be taken from Kate and Martin for chromosome analysis. The results showed that Martin carried a balanced Robertsonian translocation between chromosomes 14 and 21. The obstetrician informed the couple of the results and referred them to the clinical genetics service.

When the genetic counsellor wrote offering the couple an appointment, she indicated that she would need to take a detailed family history. Mary and her husband had moved 300 miles south to England from a small Scottish village when they were first married and had lost touch with her family.

Martin explained the need for a family history to his mother. Mary was able to track down one of her sisters, who still lived in the same village. Mary was pleased to re-establish contact with this sister and was able to obtain up-to-date information about the rest of her family.

When the GC took a detailed family history from Kate and Martin, this showed that several children in Martin's extended family had been born with Down syndrome, and there had been more miscarriages than one would normally expect.

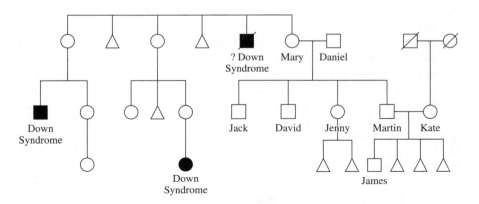

Pedigree 6.2

Ninety five percent of cases of Down syndrome are caused by non-disjunction at meiosis, resulting in three separate copies of chromosome 21. Approximately 4% are due to a balanced Robertsonian translocation between chromosome 21 and one of the other acrocentric chromosomes (13, 14, 15 and 22), resulting in three copies of chromosome 21, two of which are separate and the third a part of the chromosome translocation.

With the aid of diagrams (see Figure 6.7) the GC was able to explain to the couple the possible outcomes in future pregnancies:

1. a baby with normal chromosomes
2. a baby with a balanced Robertsonian translocation the same as Martin's
3. a baby with trisomy 21, which can result in the birth of a live baby with Down syndrome
4. a baby with trisomy 14, which would result in early miscarriage.

Kate and Martin were glad to have an explanation for their miscarriages. Previously Kate had worried that it was her 'fault', due to something that she had inadvertently done wrong while pregnant. She did not blame Martin as she felt the translocation was beyond his control. Martin had felt very guilty when he first received his results but was coming to terms with the news with help and support from Kate.

The couple was now very worried about the risk to future pregnancies. The laboratory was able to predict the likelihood of a child of Martin's being conceived with Down syndrome as <1%. Had Kate been the carrier, the risk would have been 10–15% as the sex of the carrier parent makes a significant difference to the risk (Firth & Hurst, 2005, p. 525). Kate and Martin were reassured to know that if a pregnancy did not result in miscarriage the chances of the baby having Down syndrome would be low. However, they felt that they would want a prenatal test to determine the baby's chromosomes as they would not want to continue with a pregnancy if the baby had Down syndrome. The GC discussed the prenatal tests available to them; CVS and amniocentesis (see Chapter 5).

Martin and Kate asked what the risk of James carrying the translocation was. The GC explained that as James was a normal healthy child who did not have Down syndrome, he had a 50% (1 in 2) chance of having either normal chromosomes or the balanced translocation. The GC offered to write to James's GP explaining the risk and suggesting that it was discussed with James when he was old enough to understand the implications and make a decision about being tested. This usually happens around the age of 16. The GC then went on to discuss testing the extended family. Mary already assumed that she was likely to be a carrier and had asked Martin to arrange for her to be tested. Martin's sister, Jenny, was also keen to be tested as she had had two miscarriages. His brothers both expressed interest in testing, especially David, as he and his partner were thinking of starting a family. Subsequent testing showed, as expected, that Mary carried the translocation.

David and his brother, Jack, were found to have normal chromosomes but Jenny carried the translocation. An appointment was made for Jenny and her husband to see the GC to discuss the implications of this result.

Mary was keen to pass on information about the translocation to her siblings. The GC therefore sent a letter to Mary which she could pass on to her family.

By the time all these test results were available, Kate was pregnant again. When Kate reached 14 weeks' gestation without any signs of miscarriage, the couple decided that they would request amniocentesis as they did not feel that they could cope with uncertainty for the remainder of the pregnancy. Kate and Martin did not want to know the sex of the baby and the laboratory was notified of this request when the amniocentesis was carried out. The test results showed a normal karyotype

---

Box 6.1   Letter for Patient with a Balanced Translocation to Show to Relatives

To the relatives of . . . .

  You may be aware that . . . . has an altered chromosome pattern, known as a translocation, between the . . . and . . . chromosomes [full karyotype displayed here]. This does not have any implications for his/her own health as no genetic material has been lost, gained or changed. However, it could lead to a significantly increased risk of miscarriage and in some situations to an increased risk of handicap in children.

  It is possible that you might also carry the same translocation. This can be checked easily on a blood sample (5 ml in lithium heparin).

  If you would like to discuss this further or pursue testing, we would be happy to hear from you or your doctor.

  Yours sincerely,

---

and the sex of the baby was not recorded on the laboratory report. This ensured that the staff looking after Kate during her pregnancy did not inadvertently reveal this unwanted information.

DELETIONS

A deletion involves the loss of part of a chromosome (sometimes called a partial monosomy). Deletions can cause phenotypic (physical) effects because of the loss of genes contained within the deleted chromosome segment. For a deletion to be seen in a karyotype, the amount of deleted material must be large and many genes will be affected. DNA techniques are now used to identify some deletions of genetic material that are too small to be identified through the microscope (e.g. FISH techniques and subtelomeric studies, see Chapter 4). Deletions occurring at the tip of a chromosome are known as terminal deletions. A deletion involving a chromosome breaking in several places, loss of genetic material and the rejoining of the chromosome arms is known as an interstitial deletion. Deletions may also occur as the result of an unbalanced translocation.

  The effects of a deletion will vary according to the importance of the genes within the deleted section. A small deletion of a region of chromosome containing tightly packed genes can cause much more severe problems than a larger deletion of a region of chromosome containing much less significant genetic material. Deletions will almost always cause developmental delay and there may also be physical abnormalities.

DUPLICATIONS

Duplication occurs when there is an extra copy of a segment of a chromosome. This is sometimes referred to as partial trisomy.

INVERSIONS

Inversions occur when a chromosome breaks in two places and the resulting middle portion turns around and is reinserted into the gap. Inversions are known as para-centric if the two breaks are in the same chromosomal arm, or as pericentric if the breaks occur in different arms of the same chromosome. If the breakpoints do not involve genes, they will not cause symptoms in the carrier but may lead to fertility problems and miscarriages.

MOSAICISM

'Somatic mosaicism' refers to an individual with two different cell lines which have derived from a single zygote (fertilised ovum). Chromosome mosaicism usually results from non-disjunction occurring at an early stage in embryonic cell division. Some cells will continue to divide normally, resulting in cells containing 46 chromosomes. Other cells, however, will have either 45 or 47 chromosomes.

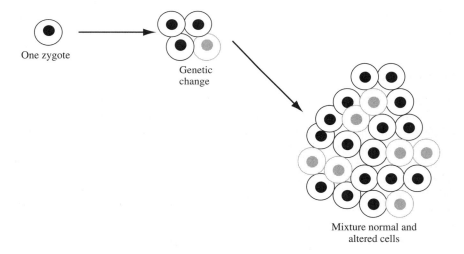

Figure 6.8 Diagram Showing Mosaicism.

Those cell lines with 45 chromosomes are unlikely to survive. If the pregnancy continues to delivery, the resulting child will have a mixture of normal and trisomic cells.

Mosaicism is found in 1–2% of children with Down syndrome. It is not possible to estimate the effect of the trisomic cells as the proportion of these cells varies in different tissues. Although it is possible to estimate the proportion of the trisomic cells in the blood and skin, the proportion in the brain cells cannot be estimated, so the degree of developmental delay that might be expected cannot be guessed at.

POINTS FOR REFLECTION

- How much information about other chromosome abnormalities should be given to a pregnant woman offered a prenatal diagnostic test to exclude Down syndrome following abnormal screening test results?
- How do you feel about termination of pregnancy for Down syndrome?
- How do you feel about termination of pregnancy for Klinefelter syndrome?
- How easy would you find it to obtain detailed information about your extended family?
- What counselling facilities are available in your area following termination of pregnancy, stillbirth or early infant death?

REFERENCES

Buchanan, A. (1997) Tinder-box criminal aggression. *The British Journal of Psychiatry*, **171**(12), 589–90.

Firth, H.V. and Hurst, J.A. (2005) *Oxford Desk Reference: Clinical Genetics*. Oxford University Press, Oxford.

Jacobs, P. *et al.* (1965) Aggressive behaviour, mental subnormality and XYY males. *Nature*, **208**, 1351–2.

7 Autosomal Dominant Disorders: 50% Risk to Offspring

JO HAYDON

Autosomal dominant conditions occur when one copy of a pair of genes is normal and the second copy is altered. The altered gene causes the individual possessing it to be affected.

A typical pedigree of a family with an autosomal dominant disorder will show:

- Affected individuals in several generations.
- Affected males and females in roughly equal proportions.
- Affected individuals with both affected and unaffected offspring.
- Transmission of the disorder by female to female or male, and by male to female or male.

Many autosomal dominant disorders are not apparent at birth but present during childhood. There are many adult-onset autosomal dominant disorders which, even within a family, have variation in the age of onset and clinical manifestations.

Various myths have developed within families about the pattern of autosomal dominant inheritance:

- **Only males or only females will be affected in the family**. When looking at the family tree, it may be that individuals of only one sex have been affected. This happens by chance, in the same way that in some families, only sons are born. This does not mean that a daughter will never be born, and neither does the fact that for generations only males have been affected mean that a female will never be affected.
- **The disease can skip a generation**. This can appear to have happened for one of two reasons. Either an individual inherited the altered gene from a parent, passed it on to a child and then died early, before they reached the age at which the disorder would have manifested itself. Alternatively, a genetic phenomenon known as reduced penetrance has occured. With reduced penetrance, the altered

gene does not always cause the disorder to occur (e.g. familial cancer, see Chapter 12). This may be because other genes have a modifying effect on the altered gene, or because the gene has been affected by environmental factors. Although the disorder appears to have skipped a generation, the gene which causes it has not.

When an individual appears to be the first in their family to be affected by a disorder, this may be due to several reasons:

- **New mutation**. When the gene mutation happens for the first time in the egg or sperm from which the individual was conceived. There is an increased risk of new dominant mutations occurring when the father is older than average at the time of conception (Mueller & Young, 2001, p. 100) (see Case Study 2).
- **Variable expression**. The genetic phenomenon whereby the same gene mutation can cause widely different effects. The effects of the gene, and thus the severity of the disease, can vary greatly within a family. When an autosomal dominant condition is diagnosed for the first time, it is important for both parents of the affected individual to be examined carefully to assess whether one of them has the same condition in a much milder form (see Case Study 3).
- **Anticipation**. The genetic phenomenon whereby a disease shows an earlier age of onset and/or more severe expression in later generations (e.g. grandfather has very mild signs, mother has moderate signs and child has severe signs). This is found in genetic disorders in which the gene mutation is caused by an unstable triplet repeat sequence. We know that within DNA the bases are arranged in triplets. Sometimes within a gene a triplet may be repeated, rather like a stutter. If the number of repeats increases beyond a certain threshold, the gene becomes altered (see Case Study 1).

When variable expression or anticipation is the reason for a genetic disorder being diagnosed in a child, and the disorder is found to be present in a parent in a milder form, the situation must be handled very carefully. The affected parent learns that they have a previously undiagnosed condition at the same time as they discover that they have passed this condtition on to their child in a more severe form. This may result in tremendous feelings of guilt.

- **Previous misdiagnosis**. With some adult onset conditions it may be that an affected parent was misdiagnosed and therefore the risk to offspring was not recognised. For example, an individual diagnosed with Huntington disease may report that one parent had Parkinson's disease or Alzheimer's disease. In retrospect, one may suspect that the parent's condition was really Huntington disease.
- **Non-paternity**. Although a possibility, this is a much less likely explanation and any suggestions of this must be handled with great tact.

If an individual is affected with an autosomal dominant disorder, each of their children will have a 1 in 2 (50%) risk of inheriting the altered gene and a 1 in 2 (50%) chance of inheriting the normal copy. When explaining this to couples, it is important that they realise that the risk applies to each individual pregnancy. Otherwise the couple may interpret the risk as meaning that alternate children will be affected/unaffected. It is often useful to describe this inheritance pattern by using the analogy of tossing a coin. Each time the coin is tossed it has an equal chance of landing heads up (affected) or tails up (unaffected). As coins have no memory, the outcome of subsequent tossings may be the same or different. Similarly, whether or not the gene is passed on is not affected by any actions on the part of the parents, e.g. smoking, drinking alcohol, etc. This may help relieve some of the feelings of guilt they will experience.

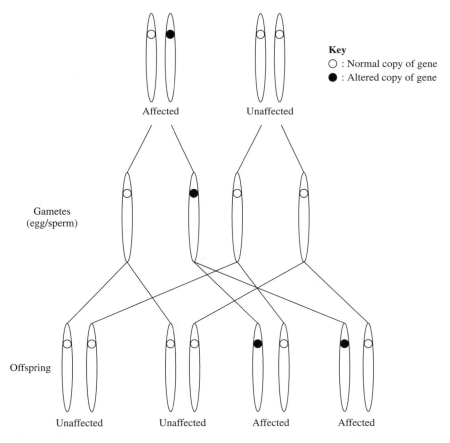

Figure 7.1 Diagram Showing Autosomal Dominant Inheritance.

If an individual inherits altered dominant genes for the same condition from both parents, this may or may not cause them to be more severely affected. In the case of achondroplasia, where two affected individuals often mate by preference, an individual who is homozygous for the condition (i.e. both of their copies of the gene are the same, and in this case altered) is likely to die early in infancy. However, an individual who is homozygous for Huntington disease does not have a more severe form of the disorder than their parents.

A new diagnosis of an autosomal dominant disorder in an individual may have implications not only for that person and their parents, but also for siblings and other members of the extended family:

- If the disorder is found to be due to a new mutation, then the risk of recurrence for the parents is eliminated and only offspring of the affected individual are at risk.

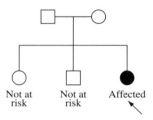

Pedigree 7.1

- If one parent is found to have a mild form of the disorder then there is a 50% risk to all of their offspring.

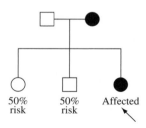

Pedigree 7.2

- If the parent of the newly diagnosed adult is thought, in retrospect, to have been affected, then there is a potential risk to a number of family members.

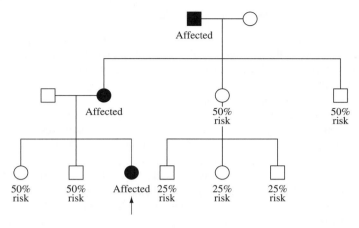

Pedigree 7.3

COMMON AUTOSOMAL DOMINANT CONDITIONS

- Achondroplasia.
- Myotonic dystrophy.
- Retinoblastoma.
- Huntington disease.
- Neurofibromatosis.
- Familial hypercholesterolemia.
- Tuberous sclerosis.
- Polycystic kidney disease.
- Osteogenesis imperfect.
- Familial adenomatous polyposis (FAP).
- Marfan's syndrome.

CASE STUDY 1: ANTICIPATION

Emily and her husband Jack were referred to the clinical genetics service several months after the death of their two-day-old daughter, Jade. This had obviously been a very traumatic time for the couple, made worse physically by Emily experiencing a post partum haemorrhage severe enough to require blood transfusion. At birth, Jade was noted to be extremely hypotonic with bilateral talipes. She also exhibited signs of severe respiratory distress and, despite treatment in the neonatal unit, died shortly afterwards. During Jade's short lifetime, the paediatrician suspected a diagnosis of congenital myotonic dystrophy and blood was taken for DNA analysis, the result of which confirmed the diagnosis.

MYOTONIC DYSTROPHY: THE DISEASE

Myotonic dystrophy is an autosomal dominant condition caused by an expansion in the gene. It is one of the commonest forms of muscular dystrophy seen in adults. There can be tremendous variation in the clinical picture due to anticipation. When the mother transmits the expanded gene, further expansion may occur, leading to the congenital form of the condition.

In the adult, clinical features include slow, progressive muscle weakness in the face and distal regions, giving rise to ptosis and a 'flat', disinterested appearance; slow relaxation of voluntary muscle after contraction (myotonia), which can be easily demonstrated by asking the affected individual to clench their fist and release it (the release will occur very slowly); early onset cataracts; frontal baldness; testicular atrophy; obstetric complications; and cardiac conduction defects. Affected individuals are also at risk when general anaesthetic is administered. Babies with the congenital form of the condition may succumb during the latter weeks of pregnancy or during labour. Those born alive will be severely hypotonic and have major respiratory and feeding problems. If they survive the neonatal period they may have marked muscle weakness and delayed development.

GENETIC COUNSELLING APPOINTMENT

Following the death of their daughter Jade, Emily and Jack received support from the bereavement counsellor attached to the obstetric unit, who helped them to start to come to terms with their loss and with the possible implications of the genetic diagnosis. When Emily and Jack felt ready to find out more about this, an appointment was made for them to see the consultant geneticist. Prior to this the couple was seen at home by the genetic counsellor, who spent some time discussing recent events, before taking a detailed family history (see Pedigree 7.4). The couple had lots of questions to ask about the condition, the risk to any future pregnancies and the implications for the extended family. The counsellor began to address these issues with them but reminded them that tests would be needed to confirm whether Emily carried the gene alteration.

During their appointment with the consultant geneticist, a neurological examination showed that Emily had early signs of muscle weakness, and a blood sample was obtained to confirm the diagnosis. Although Emily had expected this to be the case, she was still very upset as, apart from the implications for her own health, it explained why Jade had been affected and meant that future children would also be at risk.

PRENATAL TESTING

Emily and Jack were anxious to know what tests would be available in future pregnancies as they were aware of the 1 in 2 (50%) risk to future children. They were informed that a prenatal test would be available which would show whether a child had inherited the altered gene. As Emily had already had one congenitally affected child, the risk of this happening again was 40% (Harper, 2004, p. 167). However, it is not always clear on prenatal testing whether a foetus has inherited a

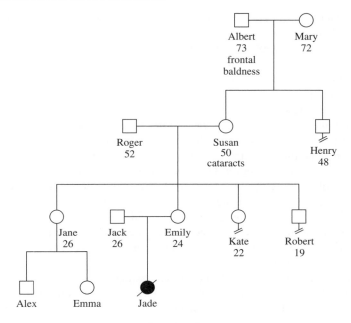

Pedigree 7.4

significantly expanded form of the gene which will result in the congenital form of the disorder. This can be a problem for some couples, who would not be concerned about a child inheriting the adult form of the disease but would wish to avoid the birth of a congenitally affected child. However, in this case Emily and Jack had already decided that they would only continue a pregnancy if the child was shown to have two normal copies of the gene. They were therefore advised to contact the genetic counsellor as soon as Emily became pregnant again so that the prenatal test could be arranged.

IMPLICATIONS FOR THE EXTENDED FAMILY

Having discussed the issues in detail, the geneticist raised the question of further family studies. Emily's mother, Susan, had a history of early onset cataract, and Susan's father had frontal baldness, both common signs of the disorder.

Emily agreed to talk to her family about the possible implications for them, and it was agreed that the GC would contact her in a few weeks' time. Following this appointment, a letter was sent to the couple summarising the information given to them. When the GC contacted Emily several weeks later, she was told that, while Emily's mother had initially been very upset to discover that she might carry the altered gene that had led to her granddaughter's death, she was keen to be tested as she had three other children and two grandchildren.

A subsequent neurological examination and DNA test confirmed that Susan was affected and she passed this information on to her other children. Susan's father had recently been diagnosed with dementia. It was felt that he was not able to give informed consent for testing. Susan's brother, Henry, was aware that he could request testing even though it had not been confirmed that he was definitely at risk. Henry declined testing at this point.

Over the next few months, Emily's sisters both underwent predictive testing. Jane already had two children but she and her partner were thinking about having a third child and wanted to know the situation before proceeding. Kate and her partner were planning to start a family in the near future and they too wanted to clarify their situation. Both sisters were found to have inherited their mother's normal copy of the gene. Emily's brother, Robert, had an initial discussion with the GC as he was unsure as to whether he wished to be tested. He was currently single, not in a relationship, and about to start the second year of his degree course. When he realised that no preventive treatment would be available if he was found to be a gene carrier he became less sure of wanting to be tested. This uncertainty was heightened when he realised the potential implications for life insurance, mortgages and employment. Robert decided to postpone testing until a later stage in his life.

Three months after the initial genetic consultation, Emily contacted the GC. This time it was to report that she was pregnant again and wanted to have a prenatal test. A dating scan and CVS were therefore arranged and a week after the test the GC was able to tell Emily that the results indicated that the baby had two normal copies of the gene. Six months later, Jack contacted the GC to let her know that their son, Ethan, was safely delivered. Although the labour had brought back painful memories for the couple, they felt that they had been able to work through the bereavement issues and were now ready to welcome their healthy son.

CASE STUDY 2: A NEW MUTATION

Janet and Philip were delighted when Janet's pregnancy was confirmed. The couple had met at a later age than average and had wondered if they might be too old to conceive. At the time of the pregnancy test Janet was 41 and Philip 50 years of age. This was Janet's first pregnancy, while Philip had two teenage daughters from a previous marriage. Because of her age, Janet requested a prenatal test. CVS showed that the baby had normal chromosomes. The remainder of the pregnancy progressed without problems and Janet had a normal delivery at term. The couple was shocked when the midwife pointed out that their son, James, had short limbs. The paediatrician confirmed this fact and a diagnosis of achondroplasia was made.

ACHONDROPLASIA: THE DISORDER

This is the commonest form of genetic short stature. The proximal limbs (humerus and femur) are shortened and the head is large, with protrusion of the frontal bones, known as frontal bossing. Intelligence and life expectancy are not affected. About 80% of children with achondroplasia are born to parents with normal height, due to a new mutation (Bonthron, 1998, p. 48).

Once Janet and Philip had had several weeks to overcome their initial shock they asked to be referred for genetic counselling.

GENETIC COUNSELLING APPOINTMENT

The geneticist obtained a family history w0hich showed, as expected, that there was no evidence of achondroplasia in either family. He explained that the condition was due to a gene alteration which appeared to have occurred for the first time when James was conceived. The couple knew that they would not be planning any further children and so were not concerned about the recurrence risk to themselves. Their

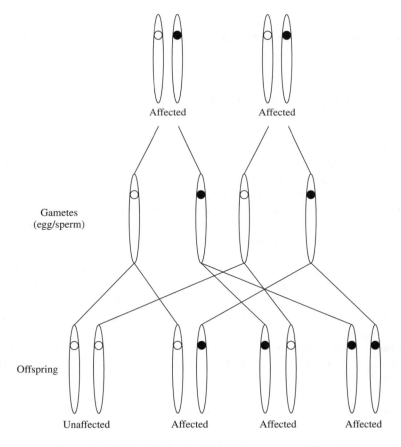

Figure 7.2 Risk to Offspring if Both Partners are Affected.

two main questions were: what was the risk to James's potential offspring and was there a risk that Philip's daughters may have children with achondroplasia?

Risk to James's Offspring

James's clinical diagnosis had been confirmed by a DNA test which showed that he had one copy of the altered gene and one normal copy. The risk to his offspring would be 1 in 2 (50%) unless his partner also had achondroplasia. In that situation the risk in each pregnancy would be 3 in 4 (75%).

If a baby inherited the altered gene from both parents (was homozygous, see Figure 7.2), this would be likely to result in the baby dying in infancy. It was suggested that James be referred for genetic counselling when he reached adulthood.

Risk to Philip's Daughters' Offspring

As Philip's daughters were unaffected, this meant that they did not carry the altered gene causing achondroplasia. The risk to their children would therefore be the same as for any individual in the general population. This risk would increase slightly if their partners were older than average but would still remain very low.

CASE STUDY 3: VARIABLE EXPRESSION

When Amjad and Mussarat took their four-year-old son, Naveed, to the accident and emergency department of their local hospital for the fourth time in three months, members of staff were initially concerned that they were dealing with a case of child abuse. Naveed's parents described him as a very active child who seemed to be accident prone, but they had also noticed that his bones fractured very easily following minor trauma. His previous injuries included fractures to both his ulna bones and his collarbone. This, his fourth fracture, was to his right tibula. The doctor examined Naveed, then asked about the family history:

- Amjad, Mussarat and their two older children had never incurred fractures.
- Both of Amjad's sisters had had a number of fractures and, indeed, one of them was now confined to a wheelchair because of multiple fractures to both legs.
- Mussarat's mother had had several fractures and so had one of her brothers, and his daughter.
- Whilst recording this information, the doctor also noticed that Amjad had blue sclera. When this was commented on, Amjad informed him that several members of both families also had this feature.

Having obtained this information, the doctor contacted the local genetics unit to confirm his suspicion that this might be osteogenesis imperfecta type 1. He was told that the signs were compatible with this diagnosis and was advised to refer the family for genetic counselling.

Naveed's fracture was set and he was to be followed up regularly at the fracture clinic until such time as the fracture had healed and the diagnosis of osteogenesis imperfecta was confirmed.

OSTEOGENESIS IMPERFECTA TYPE 1: THE DISEASE

This is an autosomal dominant condition often referred to as 'brittle bone disease'. There are four types of this condition, the commonest of which is type 1, which has the following main features:

- Bones: all bones, particularly those of the arms and legs, are fragile and prone to fractures. Fractures often happen in toddlers when they are learning to walk and have frequent falls. Osteoporosis may occur later in life.
- Eyes: the sclera (white part of the eye) may have a marked blue colouring, which persists throughout life.
- Teeth: may be discoloured (yellowish/brown), are easily cracked or broken and are prone to decay.
- Hearing: deafness may occur later in life.
- Blood vessels: may be fragile, so that bruising easily occurs.

The combination of frequent fractures and bruising may lead to an erroneous diagnosis of child abuse if a careful family history is not obtained.

GENETIC COUNSELLING

Prior to their appointment with a consultant geneticist, Amjad and Mussarat were seen by the genetic counsellor and a detailed family history was taken. Information about fractures and blue sclera was recorded and the GC asked about any history of deafness and unusually shaped teeth. The couple was surprised to be asked this until the GC explained that there was a condition that could cause all four signs and that people with the condition could have them in any combination.

When the geneticist examined Amjad and Naveed, he confirmed that they were both affected with osteogenesis imperfecta type 1. Mussarat was also examined and was found to have no clinical signs of the disorder. The geneticist, using the family tree, was able to demonstrate which of the other family members appeared to be affected. The couple expressed concern about their daughter Sagira, who had broken teeth, and it was agreed that an appointment would be made for Sagira and her brother Aziz to be seen.

The geneticist then explained the phenomenon of variable expression in simple terms as the couple was perplexed as to how the same disorder could affect family members in different ways. He also explained that although the risk to subsequent pregnancies was 1 in 2 (50%), there was no way of knowing how mildly or severely an individual would be affected.

As Amjad and Mussarat were first cousins, they wondered if this had contributed to Naveed being affected. They were reassured that this had no bearing on the

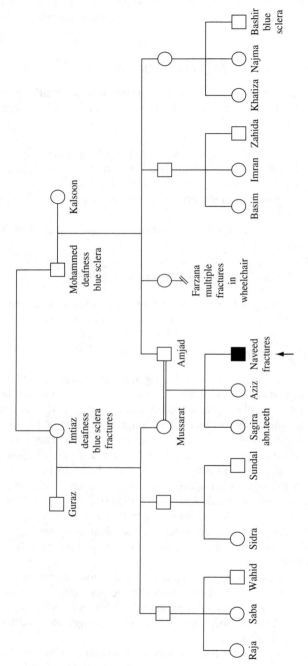

Pedigree 7.5

inheritance pattern. As Sagira appeared to be affected as well, the risk to the children of both Naveed and Sagira would be 1 in 2 (50%). If Aziz was unaffected, his children would not be at risk. If he married a first cousin, his children would only be at risk of this condition if his wife was affected herself. The couple was very relieved to hear this. They were not planning to extend their family but if a pregnancy was to occur they would not want prenatal diagnosis.

At a subsequent appointment, Sagira was found to be affected. Aziz showed no signs at present but could not be said to be definitely unaffected at this young age. It was suggested that all three children be seen again when they were young adults to answer any questions that they might have.

IMPLICATIONS FOR THE EXTENDED FAMILY

During their first appointment, Amjad and Mussarat said they would be meeting with members of their extended family later that day to discuss the information given to them by the geneticist. They were told that the genetic team would be happy to see other family members if they wanted further advice and/or a clinical examination.

Over the course of the next six months, Mussarat's brother, Shafiq, and Amjad's sister, Qamar, requested appointments. Both were found to be affected and were given similar information to Amjad and Mussarat. None of the other siblings requested appointments.

CASE STUDY 4: PREDICTIVE TESTING FOR AN UNTREATABLE CONDITION

As previously stated, many autosomal dominant disorders only present in adult life. If the gene mutation for the disorder is known, it is possible for individuals at risk of having inherited the altered gene to have a presymptomatic or predictive test (see Chapter 4) to clarify their situation.

Jordan was referred for genetic counselling by his general practitioner. Jordan's grandfather, uncle and aunt had all been diagnosed with Huntington disease (HD) and Jordan was anxious to know if he would also be affected at some time in the future.

While drawing up the family tree, the genetic counsellor discovered that Jordan's grandfather became affected at the age of 39 years and subsequently died aged 52, when Jordan was only 7 years old. Jordan had only vague memories of his grandfather, who had been in a nursing home for the last few years of his life. Jordan's uncle, Sam, had had juvenile onset HD (see below) and died before Jordan was born. His aunt, Sally, was diagnosed with the disorder two years ago but Jordan had little contact with her. Jordan's mother, Pamela, and her younger sister, Alice, had both indicated that they did not wish to know if they carried the gene for HD.

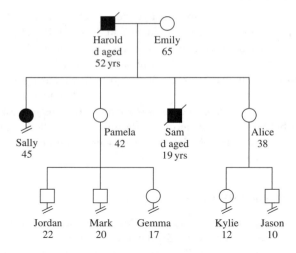

Pedigree 7.6

HUTINGTON'S DISEASE: THE CONDITION

HD is an autosomal dominant neurological disorder with variation in age of onset and manifestation:

- Physically, fidgety movements, gradually worsening in some patients, may lead to clumsiness and problems with balance and walking. Difficulties with speech and swallowing and weight loss may also become apparent as the disease progresses.
- Psychologically, depression is a common manifestation of the disorder. This may occur because the individual has realised that they are affected (reactive) but may also be an inherent aspect of the condition. An increased incidence of suicide has been found amongst affected individuals (DiMaio *et al.*, 1993). The disease may also cause irritability, leading to aggression, both verbal and (less commonly) physical.
- Cognitive function may also be affected, with the individual showing features of early-onset dementia.

The disease progresses slowly over a period of 15–20 years and the average age of onset is between 30 and 55 years. The symptoms of the disorder may be alleviated with medication to some extent but at present there is no cure. The gene mutation was identified in 1993 and was found to be due to an expansion in repeats of a triplet (CAG) within the gene. Repeats of up to 35 fall within normal limits; 37 or more repeats will give rise to the disease (although 37–39 repeats may cause very late onset of the disorder); a result of 36 repeats can be difficult to interpret. Now that the gene has been found, accurate presymptomatic testing is available to at-risk individuals. An internationally-agreed protocol for presymptomatic testing was drawn up because of the combination of the fact that there is no preventive therapy and the suicide risk associated with HD.

JUVENILE ONSET HUNTINGTON DISEASE

Occasionally the disease occurs in childhood, when it is known as juvenile HD. This happens when the gene has undergone a large expansion (60–100 repeats) and it is almost always transmitted through the father (Mueller & Young, 2001).

GENETIC COUNSELLING APPOINTMENTS

Jordan was very keen to know if he was going to develop HD when he was older. He felt that this information would help him to plan for the future. He knew that he would only be at risk if his mother had inherited the gene but this was a subject that she avoided talking about. Jordan was therefore keen to know if there was a test available to him.

PRESYMPTOMATIC TESTING: THE PROCESS

It is most important that individuals requesting this test understand the difference between a presymptomatic test and a diagnostic test. If the altered gene for HD has been inherited, it is present from the moment of conception. Diagnosis of this disorder is made on clinical findings. If an individual has no clinical signs but wishes to know if they will become affected at an unknown time in the future, a DNA test can predict this.

It is recommended that individuals have known about their risk for at least six months before preparing for the test. Often when an adult hears about the risk for the first time, the initial reaction is, 'I need to know, there is a test that will tell me, I will have the test.' However, when given time to reflect on the implications of finding out, many people decide to postpone testing until a later date.

Individuals should only be tested if the decision is theirs, and not due to coercion from another. Sometimes, understandably, partners are keen for the at-risk individual to be tested so that they can plan for the future and know if there is a risk to their offspring. The author has also known cases of pressure-to-test exerted by a judge hoping to decide the settlement in a divorce case and by a solicitor wishing to use the information following a guilty verdict in the hope that it might affect the sentence about to be handed down.

The presymptomatic testing process takes place over a period of months. The individual is seen on several occasions by members of the genetic team, including for a psychological assessment, and may have a neurological examination. During these consultations, the following issues are discussed in detail:

- The signs, symptoms and progress of the disorder.
- Variations in age of onset and length of disease.
- Autosomal dominant inheritance and the risk to the individual and other family members.
- The impact of a positive result (i.e. finding the altered gene) on the individual and on their partner, family and friends.
- Living with the knowledge that one will become affected with the condition when there is no preventive treatment and no indication of when or how the disease will present.
- Implications for life insurance and mortgages.

Consideration also needs to be given to who will be the individual's main support, e.g. partner or close friend. This person may attend the pre-test consultations with them. The results of the test are always given face to face and preferably with the support person present.

Follow-up support is offered to individuals following the test, regardless of the result. The amount of support will vary according to individual needs.

ADVANTAGES OF TESTING

- The individual's uncertainty about their gene status is removed.
- If the results show that the individual does not carry the altered gene, they know that they will not become affected and that present or potential offspring will also be unaffected.
- If the test is positive, the individual can start to plan for the future.

DISADVANTAGES OF TESTING

- A positive result removes all hope of avoiding the disorder.
- Uncertainty about gene status is clarified but is replaced with uncertainty about how and when the disorder will present.
- A positive result also confirms that any existing or future children will be at 50% risk of inheriting the disorder, although in the case of future pregnancies, prenatal testing or possibly pre-implantation diagnosis will be available.
- A negative result may lead to problems for the individual accepting their 'new identity' (i.e. no longer being at risk of developing HD) because they have lived with this threat for so long.
- Expectations of the impact of a good result on the individual's life may be unrealistic. The individual may expect that all their problems, e.g. with relationships or anger management, will disappear.
- There may be feelings of guilt because the individual has escaped the disorder while their siblings are either affected or still at risk.

JORDAN'S ISSUES

The genetic counsellor discussed all the relevant issues in detail with Jordan. It was particularly important for him to consider how he might cope with a bad result at his age (22), when it might be another 20 years or more before he would become affected. He also needed to consider how this might impact on any future relationships; at what stage in a relationship would he tell a new partner about his status and how might she react to this information? The potential risk to his offspring and the various options available were also discussed. However, the most important issue was that Jordan was not at 50% risk, as his mother's gene status was unknown. Her risk was 50% and Jordan's was half of this, i.e. 25%. This situation gives rise to another set of problems.

TESTING INDIVIDUALS AT 25% RISK

Individuals may request a presymptomatic test when they are at 25% risk either because the intervening parent has died early from some other cause or because that parent has declined testing.

If the result of Jordan's test was negative, he would know that he would not become affected, but both his mother's and his siblings' risks would remain the same. However, if Jordan's test result was positive, he would know that he would become affected at some future date and also that his mother was a gene carrier and his siblings' risks had increased from 25% to 50%. Jordan's mother had at some point indicated that she did not want to know if she carried the altered gene. She had a right not to know but Jordan had a right to know. There are two possible ways that this situation can be managed:

- Jordan could tell his mother that he was requesting the test and she would then know that his result might give him information about her that she did not want to know.
- Alternatively, he could not tell her that he was being tested. He would then have to be prepared to not disclose a bad result to anyone except his support person, as he would be divulging information not only about himself but also about his mother. He would also be unable to inform his siblings that they were at a definite 50% risk.

The GC suggested that Jordan raise the issue of testing with his mother and explain his need to know his own gene status so that she was aware of his concerns and could review her own decision. Jordan was advised to give careful consideration to all the issues that had been discussed. The GC agreed to write to him, summarising all the information given. No further action would be taken unless Jordan contacted her again to take matters forward.

Several months went by with no contact. Then the GC was contacted by Jordan's mother, Pamela, requesting an appointment to discuss the situation.

PAMELA'S DECISION

Jordan had discussed his concerns with his mother, who had not been aware of how much the uncertainty about his future health was affecting him. One of Pamela's reasons for deciding not to be tested was to protect her children from the possibility of knowing they were definitely at risk. Following a long and emotional discussion with Jordan, she had also raised the subject with her other children, Mark and Gemma. Neither of them expressed any immediate concern for themselves but both were keen that their mother made the choice that she felt most comfortable with. Having given the matter further thought, Pamela felt that she was indeed ready to know.

Pamela's husband, Steve, accompanied her for all of her pre-test consultations and was her major source of support. It quickly became apparent that the knowledge of the disorder being in the family and the possible implications for herself had had a major impact on Pamela's life. Pamela was only ten years old when her father was first diagnosed with the condition. Four years later her young brother, Sam, became affected. She had found this very difficult to cope with and spent a lot of time away from home. Sam died when she was 17 years old. She married at the age of 18 and a year later gave birth to Jordan. Pamela's father died four years later. The effect of the disorder on her life had receded a little after that time but her older sister's diagnosis two years ago brought all those painful memories to the fore again.

Pamela found the pre-test process painful, but very helpful in sorting out many of the feelings that she had carried with her for such a long time. When the results of her blood test were available, she and Steve were delighted to hear that she had not inherited the altered gene from her father and that therefore neither she nor her three children would develop the illness.

Several weeks later the GC contacted Pamela, as previously arranged. Pamela was pleased to have this contact as, after the initial euphoria following the result, she now reported feeling rather flat and empty. At a subsequent appointment, Pamela explored these feelings in more detail. She described the previous threat of HD as being 'Like having a parrot on my shoulder. He squawked in my ear and made a mess down my back and I thought I would never be rid of him. Now that he's gone, however, I find myself looking for him and grieving his loss.' The GC continued to see Pamela for the next few months until she had worked through her feelings of bereavement and guilt at having 'survived' when others in the family had not. By the end of that time, Pamela was able to enjoy the knowledge that she no longer needed to worry about herself or her children.

CASE STUDY 5: PREDICTIVE TESTING FOR A TREATABLE CONDITION

Richard was devastated when his brother, Peter, died from colon cancer at the age of 38 years. Peter had been working under a great deal of stress for some time and had attributed his weight loss, loss of appetite and change in bowel habits to that. He had been admitted to hospital with acute abdominal pain, vomiting and constipation, and an emergency laporoscopy revealed a tumour in his colon, with metastases in his liver and lung. During the operation, it was noted that he had multiple adenomatous polyps in his colon and a diagnosis of familial adenomatous polyposis (FAP) was made. Sadly, Peter's condition did not improve following surgery and one week later he died.

FAMILIAL ADENOMATOUS POLYPOSIS: THE DISEASE

This is an autosomal dominant condition which accounts for 1% of colorectal cancer. Affected individuals develop hundreds of polyps in the colon and/or rectum which will inevitably progress to malignancy if untreated. The polyps develop at a variable age from about 10–40 years. The average age of developing colorectal cancer if untreated is 39 years.

Treatment involves the removal of the large bowel, as the vast number of polyps makes it impossible to remove them one by one. There are three possible operations which may be used:

- Colectomy with ileorectal anastomosis (IRA). The whole of the colon is removed and the end of the ileum is joined to the rectum. Polyps may develop in the rectum and therefore, following this operation, patients will require six-monthly sigmoidoscopy for life.
- Panprotocolectomy with pouch. Both the colon and the rectum are wholly removed. An artificial rectum (pouch) is then made out of the lower end of the ileum. This is joined to the anus to allow normal bowel action.
- Total protocolectomy with permanent ileostomy. This involves removing the colon, rectum and anus and is very rarely needed in the treatment of FAP.

The family history revealed that Richard's mother had died from colon cancer at the age of 42 and in retrospect it was suspected that she too might have had FAP. Richard and his other siblings, Tony and Sandra, were advised to seek urgent colonoscopies because of the possibility that they too might have inherited the disorder. Tony and Sandra had normal results but Richard's colonoscopy revealed that he had hundreds of adenomatous polyps in his large bowel. He was advised to have immediate surgery before any of the polyps became malignant, and a colectomy with IRA was carried out within several weeks.

Richard made a good postoperative recovery but was extremely concerned about the possible risk to his two children, Martin, aged 12, and Sophie, aged 9. He was referred to the clinical genetics service and he asked for an appointment as soon as possible.

GENETIC COUNSELLING

The genetic counsellor visited Richard and his wife, Hilary, at their home, and found that although Richard was making good progress, the couple was extremely anxious about any risk to their children.

Having drawn up a family tree, the GC went on to explain autosomal dominant inheritance, which indicated that Martin and Sophie each had a 50% risk. The couple was very upset about this and needed reassurance that early diagnosis and treatment could give a normal life expectancy. They were anxious for the children to be seen as soon as possible. The GC explained that the management of the children would depend to some extent on whether the altered gene could be identified in Richard. An appointment was arranged for the couple to see a geneticist. A blood sample was obtained from Richard and he was warned that the results might take several months. Once Richard and Hilary knew that the children were not at imminent risk of developing bowel cancer they became more relaxed.

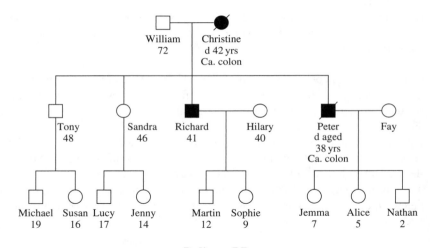

Pedigree 7.7

At the next consultation the geneticist reiterated the information about the disorder and the means of inheritance and the fact that the management of the children would depend on whether or not a mutation was found in Richard.

MUTATION SCREENING

FAP is caused by an alteration in a gene carried on chromosome 5. The gene alteration can vary from family to family. Once the mutation has been identified in an affected individual, a presymptomatic test can be offered to other family members who are at risk. Finding the mutation in the affected individual may take weeks or months.

Mutation Found

Martin would be seen as soon as his parents felt he was ready. An explanation of his situation would be given to him and a blood sample would be obtained. If this showed that he had not inherited the gene mutation, no further action would be necessary. If the mutation was found to be present, Martin would be referred to the colorectal surgeon so that the family could discuss the most appropriate time for Martin to have surgery. Some teenagers prefer this to happen before starting year 10 and their GCSE modules. Others prefer to postpone surgery until after their GCSEs or A levels. If surgery is postponed for any reason, colonoscopy will be required every six months to ensure that there are no polyps undergoing changes which might lead to early colon cancer. Martin would also be able to discuss which type of surgery might be most appropriate.

Mutation Not Found

Annual colonospy would be advised up to the age of 40 years. As one might imagine, this is quite a daunting proposition, not without risk, and not readily accepted by teenagers. As Sophie was only 9 years old, no screening would be necessary for her for another year.

Richard and Hilary were advised to think about how they would tell the children of their possible risk of developing FAP. Both children had been shocked when their father was admitted to hospital and it was felt wise to postpone telling them for a month or two. This would give them time to recover from the shock and enable Richard's progress to be an indication to them of how treatable the condition was. Within several weeks, the laboratory found the mutation in Richard. By this time the couple had talked with Martin, who was mature for his age and wanted to clarify his situation as soon as possible.

MARTIN'S CONSULTATION

Martin was a remarkably mature young boy who had had some genetic lessons in his biology course. He quickly grasped his 50% risk and the fact that this could be clarified with a blood test, which he was keen to proceed with. This subsequently showed that he had not inherited the mutation and so no further screening was required. Sophie would be due for an appointment in one year's time. Her name was entered onto the computer system so that a reminder would be given to the geneticist when this appointment was due.

THE EXTENDED FAMILY

Richard also raised the issue of the risk with his late brother's children. Peter had left three young children aged 7, 5 and 2. His wife, Fay, had indicated her concern about the children but was struggling to cope with her own grief, that of the children and the practicalities of suddenly becoming a single parent. She was aware that no testing would be offered to the children at that stage and it was agreed that she would contact the GC when she was ready to find out more.

Two months later, Fay contacted the GC and a home visit was arranged. After spending some time discussing bereavement issues, the GC moved on to discuss FAP and the implications for the children. Fay was relieved to know that it would be another three years before the oldest girl, Jemma, would be offered an appointment as she felt this would give her daughter time to recover from the loss of her father.

The GC emphasised how important it was that the children were seen when they were old enough as FAP is a treatable condition. It was agreed that their GP be notified that each child should be offered an appointment when they reached the age of 10 years. Fay also agreed to them being registered on the genetic database, which would remind the geneticist when the children were due for an appointment. The approach to families with FAP is much more proactive than for families with Huntington disease because there is a treatment available which can avoid early death.

POINTS FOR REFLECTION

- In families with autosomal dominant conditions there may be a number of affected individuals in several generations. This may mean that the family is too busy caring for the affected individuals to access the help it needs.
- Affected individuals within the same family may make very different decisions about the options available to them.
- Affected individuals within the same family may experience the condition with varying degrees of severity.
- The professional dealing with several individuals within the same family must respect each of these individuals' confidentiality.
- How might you raise the issue of non-paternity?

REFERENCES

Bonthron, D. *et al.* (1998) *Clinical Genetics: A Case-based Approach*, W.B. Saunders, London.

DiMaio, L. (1993) Suicide risk in Huntington disease. *Journal of Medical Genetic*, **30**(4), 289–92.

Harper, P.S. (2004) *Practical Genetic Counselling*, 6th edn, Arnold, London.

Mueller, R.F. and Young, I.D. (2001) *Emery's Elements of Medical Genetics*, 11th edn, Churchill Livingstone, London.

8 Autosomal Recessive Disorders: Unaffected Parents with 25% Risk to Offspring

JO HAYDON

Autosomal recessive conditions occur when both copies of a gene pair are altered. It is the absence of a normal copy of the gene that causes an individual to be affected, rather than the 'double dose' of the altered gene. One normal copy of the gene is sufficient for adequate cell function. An individual with two altered copies of the gene will always be affected as these disorders are fully penetrant. There is usually very little clinical variability within families.

A typical pedigree of a family with an autosomal recessive disorder will show:

- Two or more affected individuals in a single sibship (i.e. brothers and sisters) within the family.
- Males and females affected equally.
- Affected individuals born to unaffected parents, who are usually unaware that they are carriers for that genetic condition.

Many autosomal recessive disorders are not apparent at birth. They are often severe, with a poor prognosis. Many inborn errors of metabolism follow this pattern of inheritance. Affected individuals may make normal progress in the first months of life before showing signs of delayed development or even regression. There may be some delay in diagnosis because there is no known family history. Along with the shock of a diagnosis which may have a poor prognosis for their child, parents have to come to terms with the fact that this is a genetic condition and that they must be carriers. Furthermore, their other existing children may be affected and there is a risk to any future children.

Such a diagnosis often leads to feelings of denial and guilt. A frequently asked question at this time is, 'How can it be inherited if no one else in the family is affected?' When an explanation is given, parents are often overwhelmed with feelings of guilt on discovering that they are both carriers for the condition. It is

Genetics in Practice: A clinical approach for healthcare practitioners   Edited by Jo Haydon
© 2007 John Wiley & Sons, Ltd

important to stress that we are all carriers for several recessive disorders (out of about 23,000 pairs of genes) but that this only causes potential problems if our partner is also a carrier. A carrier is an individual with one normal copy of the gene and one altered copy and would be expected to be healthy. Parents who have a common ancestor are more likely to be carriers for the same condition. Recessive disorders are therefore more common in consanguineous relationships, i.e. where partners are related by blood.

If both members of a couple are carriers for the same recessive disorder, there are four possible outcomes each time conception occurs, because in each egg or sperm there is an equal chance (1 in 2 or 50%) that there will be a normal copy or an altered copy of the gene:

- Both individuals pass on the normal copy of the gene and the child therefore has a normal pair of genes and is unaffected.
- The male partner passes on his normal copy of the gene and the female passes on her altered copy. The child is therefore normal as they have a normal copy of the gene, but is a carrier for the condition.
- The male partner passes on his altered copy of the gene and the female passes on her normal copy. Once again, the child is normal as they have a normal copy of the gene, but is a carrier for the condition.
- Both parents pass on the altered copy of the gene and the child is therefore affected as they do not have a normal copy of the gene.

When explaining this to couples it is important to ensure that they understand that this 1 in 4 (25%) risk applies to each individual pregnancy. Otherwise the couple may interpret the risk as meaning that as they have one affected child the next three will be unaffected. It is useful to describe this inheritance pattern by using the analogy of tossing two coins. Each time the two coins are tossed simultaneously there are four possible combinations of the way they fall. Provided at least one coin lands tails up, the child will be unaffected. As coins have no memory, the outcome of subsequent tossings may be the same or different. Similarly, whether the couple's future offspring is affected or unaffected does not depend on any actions on the part of the parents, e.g. smoking, drinking alcohol, etc. This may help to relieve some of the feelings of guilt experienced by the parents.

Diagnosis of an autosomal recessive disorder in a child does not only have implications for the immediate nuclear family (parents and siblings) but also for members of the extended family. It is likely that the gene mutation for the disorder has been present in the family for many generations. It may not have been recognised previously because carriers have, by chance, chosen partners who are not carriers for the same disorder. Even if two carriers have had children together, with each pregnancy they had a 3 in 4 (75%) chance of having a child who was not affected. When the diagnosis is made, a numerical risk can be assigned to individuals within the family. If the population carrier risk for the disorder is also known, couples can be given an estimated risk of having an affected child.

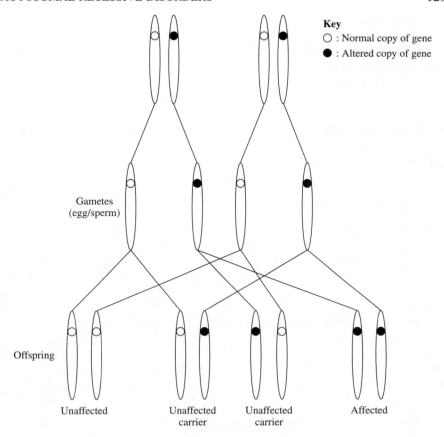

Figure 8.1 Diagram Showing Autosomal Recessive Inheritance.

COMMON AUTOSOMAL RECESSIVE CONDITIONS

- Congenital adrenal hyperplasia
- Cystic fibrosis
- Freidrieck's ataxia
- Haemochromatosis
- Haemoglobinopathies including:

  1. Beta Thalassaemia
  2. Sickle cell disease

- Sensori-neural deafness
- Spino-Muscular Atrophy (SMA)
- Zellweger syndrome
- Inborn errors of metabolism including:

1. Galactosaemia
2. Hemocystinuria
3. Mucopolysaccaridoses
4. Phenylketonuria
5. Tay Sachs disease

ESTIMATING RISK

BROWN/HOOPER FAMILY

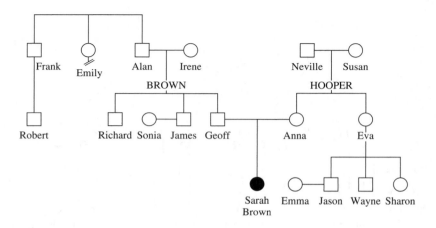

Pedigree 8.1

Imagine that Sarah Brown has been diagnosed with an autosomal recessive disorder and that the population carrier frequency for this disorder is 1 in 40.

Her father, Geoff, and her mother, Anna, are obligate carriers (i.e. they must be carriers).

Geoff's brother, James, has a 1 in 2 risk of being a carrier as either Alan or Irene must be a carrier.

James's partner, Sonia, has a population risk of 1 in 40 of being a carrier.

Therefore the risk to James and Sonia of having a child affected with the same condition as Sarah is: $(1 \text{ in } 2) \times (1 \text{ in } 40) \times (1 \text{ in } 4) = 1 \text{ in } 320$ (i.e. $\sim 0.33\%$).

Anna's older sister, Eva, has a 1 in 2 risk of being a carrier as either Neville or Susan must be a carrier.

Eva's oldest son, Jason, has half his mother's risk of being a carrier, i.e. 1 in 4. Jason's partner, Emma, has a population risk of 1 in 40 of being a carrier.

Therefore the risk to Jason and Emma of having a child affected with the same condition as Sarah is: $(1 \text{ in } 4) \times (1 \text{ in } 40) \times (1 \text{ in } 4) = 1 \text{ in } 640$ (i.e. $\sim 0.16\%$).

IS FURTHER CLARIFICATION POSSIBLE?

It may be possible to clarify the risks further in this family. If the gene mutation in Sarah's family is known, or if carrier status can be clarified by haematological tests (for haemoglobinopathies) or enzyme assay (for metabolic disorders), it may be possible to determine individual family member's carrier status. This knowledge would refine the risk for individual couples.

If James is not a carrier there is no risk to his offspring.

However, if he is a carrier, the risk to James and Sonia of having an affected child is: $1 \times (1$ in $40) \times (1$ in $4) = 1$ in 160 (i.e. it has doubled but is still below 1%).

If the test that clarified the family members' carrier status could also be used on individuals who do not have a family history of the condition, even more clarification would be possible.

Let's imagine Sonia and Emma can also be tested to determine whether or not they were carriers.

If both James and Sonia are found to be carriers, they have a 1 in 4 risk of having an affected child. If one is found to be a carrier but the other is not, their children would not be affected but would each have a 1 in 2 risk of being a carrier. If neither James nor Sonia are carriers there is no risk of their having either affected or carrier children. The same applies to Jason and Emma when both their results are known.

When carrier testing is available within a family with an autosomal recessive disorder, a logical system of testing known as cascade screening is employed. In the first instance in the Brown family, carrier testing would be offered to Geoff and Anna's parents and siblings, each of whom has a 1 in 2 risk of being a carrier. The implications of the results will vary and this needs to be considered when arranging carrier testing. We can consider some of the individuals who could be offered testing and how they might react.

- **Richard** (Geoff's brother) is currently single and does not have a partner. He may feel it would be more appropriate to wait until he is in a stable relationship and planning a family before considering carrier testing. He and his partner could then be seen and offered testing simultaneously.
- **James** (Geoff's other brother) is married to Sonia and they plan to start a family in the near future. The diagnosis in Sarah and its implications for them has caused them a great deal of anxiety. If carrier tests are available they may wish to be tested as soon as possible so that if they are both carriers they can investigate the possibility of prenatal testing before embarking on a pregnancy.
- **Eva** (Anna's older sister) does not plan to have further children but her oldest son, Jason, is in a stable relationship. Eva may want to know her carrier status so that she can help to clarify Jason's risk. She may also want to know if her other children, Wayne and Sharon, are at risk of being carriers so that she can discuss this with them.
- **Alan** (Geoff's father) may want to know if he is a carrier. He realises that if he is a carrier he may feel guilty that the gene alteration passed by him to his son has

contributed to his granddaughter being affected. He may also worry about the possibility that his other children are carriers. However, if he is a carrier he will be able to warn his brother, Frank, whose son is planning to start a family soon. Alan may not be as worried about his sister, Emily, as she has no offspring.

Once carrier testing has clarified which of Sarah's grandparents are carriers, their siblings can also be offered carrier testing. Then, in turn, the offspring of any carriers can be tested. In a large extended family there may be a number of individuals to be tested and it may take several months before all those at-risk individuals wishing to be tested can obtain their results.

CASE STUDY 1: DIAGNOSIS OF CYSTIC FIBROSIS IN A RELATIVE

Jane's GP referred her to the clinical genetics service when her nine-month-old nephew, Richard, was diagnosed with cystic fibrosis (CF). Jane and her partner, Philip, have one son, Jack, aged 2 years, and wanted to know if he might be affected, and also if there was a risk to any future children they might have.

An appointment was arranged for them to see the genetic counsellor. The GC began the consultation by clarifying what Jane and Philip hoped to achieve during the appointment and then obtained a detailed family history from them. The couple knew very little about the disease, so the GC spent some time explaining the condition and the nature of autosomal recessive inheritance.

CYSTIC FIBROSIS: THE DISEASE

Cystic fibrosis is an autosomal recessive disease caused by an altered gene which makes gland secretions thicker or more viscous than normal. The main effect is thick bronchial mucous, causing a tendency to chest infections from childhood, increasing as the individual gets older. This can lead to progressive damage and failure of the lungs, when transplantation will be required. Thick secretions also affect the pancreas, which fails to secrete the digestive enzymes required to break down food for absorption. Consequently, children and adults may have difficulty in absorbing fatty substances and protein, causing growth failure and late physical development. Taking enzyme supplements in tablet form can help with this problem. Meconium ileus, which is obstruction of the small intestine due to excessively thick meconium, may occur in the newborn and requires surgery. Affected individuals will go through puberty, although this may be late. Women with cystic fibrosis are normally fertile, whereas affected men are nearly always infertile due to blockage or absence of the sperm ducts. Sexual function is otherwise completely normal and affected males can seek treatment using IVF techniques. Diabetes becomes increasingly frequent as patients get older.

Treatment of cystic fibrosis includes physiotherapy two or three times a day for life. Enzyme supplements are needed to aid digestion. Antibiotic treatment is commenced at the earliest sign of infection and continued longer than would be required by an otherwise healthy individual. Affected individuals may need to be admitted to hospital regularly throughout life to deal with problems as they present. Although the lifespan of affected individuals has improved with new treatments, the disease remains potentially lethal throughout life.

The GC was able to use the family pedigree to explain the likelihood of Jane, and several of her family members, being carriers.

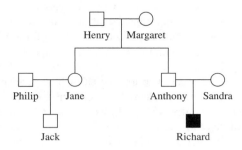

Pedigree 8.2

- Jane's brother, Anthony, and his partner, Sandra, are obligate carriers (i.e. must be carriers) as their son is affected. Each time they have a child together there is a 1 in 4 risk of the child being affected.
- Anthony has inherited the gene mutation from one of his parents, therefore Jane has a 1 in 2 risk of being a carrier.
- Philip's risk of being a carrier is the population risk for his ethnic group. As Philip is a Northern-European Caucasian, this is 1 in 25.

Therefore the risk to Jane and Philip of having an affected child is: 1 in 2 (Jane's risk) X 1 in 25 (Philip's risk) X 1 in 4 (the risk for two carriers) = 1 in 100 (50%).

This risk can be clarified further by testing Jane and Philip for CF mutations.

GENETIC TESTING FOR CYSTIC FIBROSIS

The CF gene is a large one and to date over 1000 different mutations have been found within it, and amongst Northern-European Caucasians, 31 of the common mutations account for 87% of gene alterations (Firth & Hurst, 2005, p. 292). When a child is clinically diagnosed with CF, DNA analysis will usually reveal the gene mutations causing the disorder. If the mutation is the same in both copies of the gene then both parents carry the same mutation. If the mutation is different in each copy, testing the parents will clarify which mutation each parent carries. This information will be necessary when offering to test members of the extended families. When both mutations are not found in a clinically affected child, testing for rarer mutations will be required at the molecular laboratory in Manchester and this may take several months.

When the mutation carried by both parents is known, prenatal diagnosis can be offered.

INTERPRETING THE RESULTS

Within a family known to carry a specific mutation for CF, if a family member does not carry that mutation they have a very low risk of being a carrier as it is highly unlikely that a different mutation would be found within the same family.

If a Northern-European Caucasian individual with no family history of CF does not carry the commonest CF mutations, their residual risk of being a carrier is reduced to less than 1 in 100 but cannot be completely excluded. Individuals from other ethnic groups will have an even lower risk of being carriers.

When only one partner is shown to be a carrier then prenatal testing is not appropriate, even if there is a residual risk, as a mutation that was not recognised in an adult would not be recognised in a foetus.

Anthony had told Jane that he had been shown to carry the delta F508 mutation (the commonest CF mutation found in Northern-European Caucasians). The laboratory would look for this mutation in Jane, along with the other common mutations. As Philip had no family history of CF, he would also be tested for the commonest mutations. Jane and Philip, like many individuals, found the concept of different mutations causing the same condition quite difficult to grasp. The GC explained it thus:

- A gene is an instruction for part of the body to carry out a particular function. Imagine that the instruction is: 'get the red cat off the mat'.
- There are a number of ways that this instruction can be altered so that its meaning becomes unclear, e.g.

  'get the ted cat off the mat' (only one letter of the instruction is changed)
  'get the red the mat' (several words are missing)
  'get the fat red cat off the mat' (a word has been added).

- It does not matter what the altered form of the instruction says. What is relevant is the fact that it is not the correct instruction.
- Knowing what the altered form says is important in testing other family members or prenatal testing.

Following this explanation, Jane and Philip felt that they had a clearer understanding of the test that was being offered and agreed to have a blood sample taken. They were told that the results would be ready within a few weeks and it was agreed that they would be notified by telephone.

The results of the tests showed that Jane was a carrier of the delta F508 mutation but that Philip did not carry any of the common mutations for CF. This reduced the risk to any future pregnancies to: 1 (Jane's risk) X $\sim$ 1 in 100 (Philip's reduced risk) X 1 in 4 =$\sim$ 1 in 400 (i.e. $\sim$ 0.25%).

However, their son Jack had a 1 in 2 risk of being a carrier, as would any future children the couple might have. During the consultation, the GC had explained that if this was the case it was important that Jack and any future children were offered carrier testing when they were old enough to understand the implications, usually at around the age of 16 years. The GC obtained permission to write to Jack's GP recommending this. She also wrote to Jane and Philip summarising all the information given to them and confirming their results.

CASE STUDY 2: UNEXPECTED DIAGNOSIS FOR BETA THALASSAEMIA MAJOR IN A CHILD

Waheeda and Safia presented at clinic several months after the diagnosis of beta thalassaemia major had been made in their fourth child, Usma. On first learning of the diagnosis, prognosis and treatment that Usma was likely to need, they had been very upset and unable to think about the genetic implications of having a child with an autosomal recessive disorder. Now that they had had several months to come to terms with the diagnosis, the paediatrician felt they were ready to find out more about the genetic implications for themselves and other family members. It is important to ensure that genetic information is given at a time when individuals are able to cope with it.

BETA THALASSAEMIA: THE DISORDER

Beta thalassaemia is an autosomal recessive disease which causes the red blood cells to contain less haemoglobin and be fewer in number.

Affected individuals born with severe beta thalassaemia major (about 90% of affected individuals) will be normal at birth but develop a severe anaemia in the first year of life. This may present as failure to thrive, with irritability, sleepiness, stunted growth and an enlarged liver. Death will occur in childhood without treatment. Treatment is with regular blood transfusions about every four to six weeks. However, this leads to an iron overload, which can damage the heart, liver, kidney and other organs. Damage to the pituitary may result in delayed puberty. Iron therefore has to be removed by drugs called iron-chelating agents. The commonest of these is desferrioxamine, which is given by subcutaneous infusion overnight by use of a pump, on five to seven nights per week from the age of 2 years. Alternatively, it can be given by intravenous infusion, continuously for seven days, followed by a seven day interval. This is an extremely burdensome treatment, and as children grow older they are more likely to object to it. A new oral treatment, Deferiprone, is currently being given in combination with subcutaneous desferrioxamine. It is hoped that it may become possible to wean children off the subcutaneous form so that only oral treatment is needed. This has the potential to dramatically improve the quality of life of affected children. A 'cure' can be effected with bone marrow transplantation if a suitable donor can be found.

At the time of the appointment, Usma was well and his parents were more relaxed with him. The genetic counsellor obtained a family history and, on drawing up the pedigree, became aware that Waleed and Safia were first cousins.

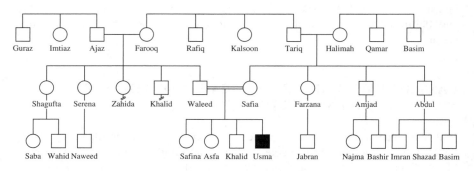

Pedigree 8.3

Waleed and Safia had completed their family and Safia was waiting to be sterilised. Even in the event of an unplanned pregnancy, the couple stated that they would not wish to consider prenatal diagnosis. Their main questions related to the risks to their other children and potential grandchildren. Members of the extended family also wanted to find out more about the likelihood of being carriers and having affected children.

The GC was able to inform Waleed and Safia that their three unaffected children each had a 2 in 3 risk of being a carrier for thalassaemia. Waleed and Safia are both carriers of a gene mutation for thalassaemia, so each time they conceive a child there is a:

- 1 in 4 risk of having an affected child.
- 2 in 4 chance of having a healthy child who is a carrier.
- 1 in 4 chance of having a healthy child who is not a carrier (see Figure 8.1).

As their first three children are unaffected, one of the four possibilities (i.e. that of being affected) has been eliminated. Of the remaining three possibilities, two are that a child will be a carrier, hence there is a 2 in 3 risk of their being a carrier. However, this would only present a problem if the carrier chose a partner who was also a carrier.

Waleed and Safia hoped that their children would marry within the family and asked the GC's advice about how they could avoid choosing a partner who was also a carrier. To answer this question it was important to establish which of their parents were carriers. Both sets of parents agreed to being tested and this was arranged through their GPs.

The results showed that Safia's father, Tariq, was a carrier but that her mother, Halimah, was not. Waleed's mother, Farooq, was a carrier but his father, Ajaz, was not. This was not surprising as Tariq and Farooq are brother and sister and must have inherited the mutation from one of their parents.

It was now possible to advise Waleed and Safia that if they chose partners for their children from either Ajaz or Halimah's extended family, they would be less likely to be carriers. In any event, when the time came for their children to marry, carrier testing could be offered to them and their chosen partner.

Carrier testing was also offered to Waleed and Safia's siblings, who all agreed to testing. Several more carriers were detected in this way, and their partners were also offered testing. Permission was obtained to notify the GPs of all the young children of the carriers so that they could be offered advice and testing when they were older, around 16 years of age. No other members of the family currently lived in the UK.

CARRIER STATUS: TESTING AND IMPLICATIONS

Carrier status is determined by haematological tests which measure serum ferritin and Hb A2. The mean corpuscular volume (MCV) and mean corpuscular haemoglobin (MCH) levels will both be reduced. This may lead to a mild anaemia, which will not usually have any effect on general health. However, it may be confused with iron deficiency anaemia. Iron therapy should not be given unless iron deficiency is found on serum iron and serum ferritin testing as otherwise iron overload could occur.

If a couple are both found to be carriers and indicate that they will want prenatal diagnosis in any future pregnancies, a sample of blood in EDTA is sent to the molecular laboratory in Oxford for mutation analysis. Mutations may vary according to ethnic origin and precise information about origin should be included on the request form.

CASE STUDY 3: UNEXPECTED CARRIER DETECTION OF SICKLE CELL DISORDER IN PREGNANCY

Marcia's parents emigrated from Jamaica to England several years before she was born. At Marcia's first antenatal clinic appointment in her third pregnancy she was offered a carrier test for sickle cell disease, which she agreed to have. Her two previous pregnancies had resulted in miscarriages at around eight weeks' gestation, before she had even attended an antenatal clinic. A week after her test, Marcia was surprised to receive a telephone call from her community midwife informing her that she was a carrier and suggesting that her partner, Craig, should also be tested.

When Craig's result showed that he was also a carrier the couple was naturally concerned and wanted more information about the risk to their pregnancy and the options available to them. They were therefore referred to the clinical genetics service for an urgent appointment and were seen by the genetic counsellor the following day.

GENETIC COUNSELLING

Marcia and Craig were very anxious when they arrived for their appointment and wanted to know as much as possible as quickly as possible. The GC explained that she wanted to begin by obtaining a family history from the couple and would then tell them about the disease, how it was inherited, the risk to their baby and the options available to them. By giving a clear outline of what was to happen during the consultation, she made the couple aware that their questions would be answered. By starting with the family history, the GC felt she would allow the couple time to relax so that when she began giving them information they would be able to take it in.

Having taken the family history, which showed, as expected, no known affected individuals in either family, the GC then described the possible effects of sickle cell disease.

SICKLE CELL: THE DISORDER

Sickle cell disorders are a group of autosomal recessive disorders in which an individual has inherited two altered copies of genes responsible for haemoglobin production. The abnormal haemoglobin produced causes red blood cells to change from their normal disc-like shape to a sickle shape (long, curved and pointed) when they are short of oxygen. These cells then become jammed in small blood vessels, blocking the blood supply and causing pain (known as a sickle cell crisis). The risk of sickling in affected individuals can be reduced by ensuring good hydration and avoiding extremes of heat and cold, stress and infection. Sickle cell crises are disruptive to normal life as they can affect schooling, employment, etc.

About a third of affected individuals have only a few medical problems. However, the disease can lead to strokes in children, to leg ulcers in adults and to damage to bones, joints, eyesight or kidneys. There is an increased incidence of premature death.

The GC explained autosomal recessive inheritance with the use of a diagram, and Marcia and Craig were able to see that there was a 1 in 4 risk to their baby. They were stunned by this news. Up until two weeks previously they had been happy and excited about the pregnancy and looking forward to the birth of their baby. Their anxieties had focused on the possibility of another miscarriage but once Marcia had reached the 10th week of the pregnancy they had begun to relax and enjoy it. Now they were aware that there was a significant risk that their baby could have a sickle cell disorder.

The next issue that they wished to discuss was the options available to them. The first option was to be aware of the risk but continue with the pregnancy. The second option was to have a prenatal test, either chorionic villus sampling (CVS) or amniocentesis (see Chapter 5). The GC explained the tests in detail, telling the couple that if they chose CVS, the test could be arranged within the next few days, while an amniocentesis could be arranged for two weeks' time. However, there were two important points for the couple to consider: first, there was a miscarriage rate of 0.5–2%, depending on which test they chose; second, as Marcia was already 14 weeks pregnant, if the results of the test showed that the baby was affected and the couple opted for termination of pregnancy, Marcia would have to have a medical termination. The couple was shocked by this news and felt that they needed to think about the situation carefully. It was agreed that the GC would telephone them in two days' time to find out what they had decided. She also gave them an information sheet about sickle cell disorder to take away with them.

When the GC spoke to Marcia two days later, she was informed that the couple had decided not to proceed with a prenatal test in this pregnancy. They felt that, having experienced two miscarriages already, they did not want a test that might cause a third one to occur, especially as the baby had a 3 in 4 chance of not being affected. Marcia also felt that she could not contemplate terminating a pregnancy at this stage. However, Marcia and Craig were anxious to know how soon after birth the baby could be tested. The GC explained that neonatal screening for sickle cell was offered to all babies in the newborn period. As Marcia's baby had a 1 in 4 risk of being affected, the GC would alert the screening laboratory, giving them Marcia's details and the expected date of delivery.

The couple felt happier about their situation now that they had reached their decision and knew that the baby could be tested soon after birth. They were also keen to tell their siblings about their risk of being carriers, and the GC agreed to send Marcia and Craig a letter which they could show to family members. If any of them then wished to be tested they could contact the local haemoglobinopathy counsellors, who would arrange screening.

CARRIER STATUS: TESTING AND IMPLICATIONS

Carrier status is determined by haematological tests, in which the common sickle cell disorders are looked for. Carriers of sickle cell should inform the anaesthetist if a general anaesthetic is required, as they are at risk of sickling if they become unusually hypoxic. They should also be advised to avoid unpressurised aircraft or deep sea diving (Firth & Hurst, 2005).

Carriers of sickle cell disorders will carry the same mutation. If both members of a couple are found to be carriers and undergo prenatal testing, a sample of blood in EDTA from each parent will be sent with the prenatal sample to the molecular laboratory in Oxford for mutation analysis.

Box 8.1   Haemoglobin Variants

There are over 800 haemoglobin variants, which may be inherited in a number of combinations, e.g. HbS, HbC, HbD Punjab, HbD not Punjab, Beta-thal.

Other variants, in combination with the sickle haemoglobin, can cause a sickle cell disorder, e.g. HbSC, HbS/beta-thal, HbS/D Punjab.

A useful web site where you can check to see whether a combination of haemoglobin variants causes a disorder is www.chime.ucl.ac.uk/APoGI

POINTS FOR REFLECTION

- How might you feel if you discovered that you carried an autosomal recessive gene mutation?
- Individuals often find it hard to accept that being a carrier for an autosomal recessive condition has no effect on their own health, and may also feel stigmatised by this status.
- How important is it to offer carrier testing to the extended family? What might this depend on?

REFERENCE

Firth, H.V. and Hurst, J.A. (2005) *Oxford Desk Reference: Clinical Genetics*, Oxford University Press, Oxford.

9 X-Linked Disorders: Carrier Mothers, Affected Sons

JO HAYDON

X-linked recessive conditions occur when an altered gene lies within the X chromosome. Males have one X chromosome and one Y chromosome, whereas females have two X chromosome. Males therefore only have one copy of each of the genes located on the X chromosome and if one of these is altered the male carrying the altered gene will be affected with whichever disorder the gene codes for. As a general rule, females who carry an altered copy of the gene will not be affected as they also carry a normal copy of that gene, which is sufficient for adequate cell function.

A typical pedigree of a family with an X-linked recessive condition will show:

- Two or more affected males in several generations.
- Females are unaffected.
- Affected males are linked through unaffected females.
- Male to male transmission does not occur.

Female carriers have a 1 in 4 risk of having an affected son because:

- They have a 1 in 2 chance of having a male or female child.
- If they are carrying a male child there is a 1 in 2 risk that he will be affected.

Also, if they are carrying a female child there is a 1 in 2 risk that she will be a carrier.

An affected male will have unaffected sons because they must inherit his Y chromosome. However, all his daughters will be obligate carriers as he will pass on his X chromosome with the altered gene to them. As they will inherit an X chromosome with a normal copy of the gene from their mother, they will be unaffected (unless she was a carrier for the same condition).

Therefore, all his children will be unaffected but any grandsons born to his daughters will have a 1 in 2 risk of being affected.

Genetics in Practice: A clinical approach for healthcare practitioners   Edited by Jo Haydon
© 2007 John Wiley & Sons, Ltd

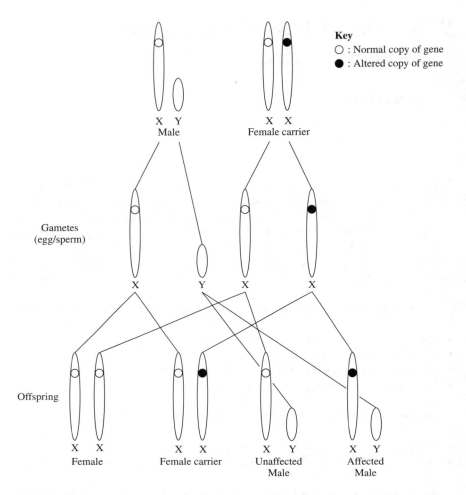

Figure 9.1 Diagram Showing X-Linked Recessive Inheritance – Female Carrier.

COMMON X-LINKED RECESSIVE CONDITIONS

- Anhidrotic ectodermal dysplasia.
- Androgen insensitivity syndrome.
- Becker's muscular dystrophy,
- Duchenne muscular dystrophy.
- Fragile X syndrome.
- Glucose 6-phosphate dehydrogenase deficiency.
- Haemophilia A & B.
- Hunter's syndrome.

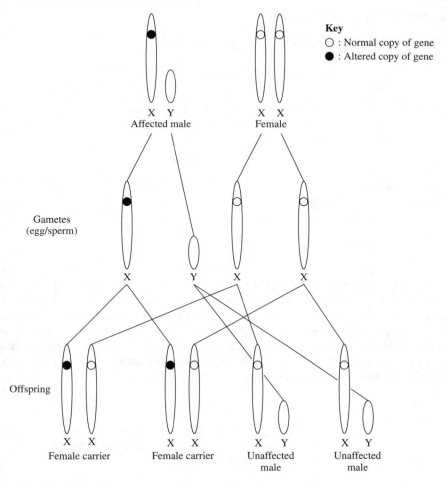

Key
○ : Normal copy of gene
● : Altered copy of gene

Figure 9.2 Diagram Showing X-Linked Recessive Inheritance – Affected Male.

- Hydrocephalus (some forms of).
- Lowe's syndrome.
- Mental retardation (some forms of).
- Occular albinism.

COMMON QUESTIONS

When a boy is diagnosed with an X-linked recessive condition, a number of questions will be raised related to the inheritance:

IS THE MOTHER A CARRIER?

A detailed family history may answer this question.

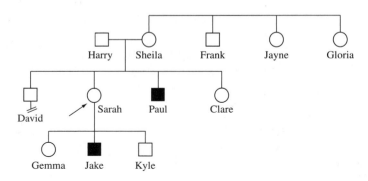

Pedigree 9.1

Sarah has an affected brother, Paul, and an affected son, Jake (Pedigree 9.1). The chance of them both being affected due to a new mutation would be exceedingly small. Therefore, one can assume that both Sarah and her mother (who has had an affected son and a carrier daughter) are carriers. Sarah's younger son, Kyle, is at risk of being affected; he may carry the altered gene but be too young to manifest signs of the condition. There are also implications for Sarah's daughter, Gemma, her sister, Clare, and her maternal aunts, Jayne and Gloria.

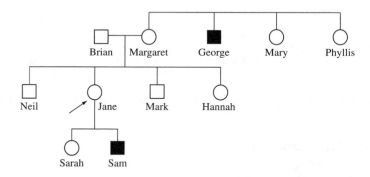

Pedigree 9.2

Jane has an affected son, Sam, and an affected maternal uncle, George (Pedigree 9.2). The chance of them both being affected due to a new mutation is extremely low and this pedigree suggests that Jane, her mother, Margaret, and her maternal grandmother are all carriers. This will have implications for Jane's daughter, Sarah, her sister, Hannah, and her maternal aunts, Mary and Phyllis.

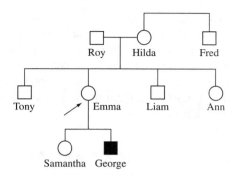

Pedigree 9.3

The disorder has presented for the first time in George (Pedigree 9.3) and may have occurred as a new mutation. It will be important to try to establish whether this arose in the egg from which George was conceived or whether Emma is a carrier. If tests show that Emma is a carrier then the risk to her offspring will follow the normal pattern and her daughter, Samantha, will have a 1 in 2 risk of also being a carrier. Further family studies will be necessary to determine if she has inherited the mutation from either of her parents.

If the tests show that she is not a carrier, this does not mean that there is no risk to any future sons. It is possible that the new mutation arose in one of Emma's egg cells early in her embryonic life and that all the cells derived from that cell will also carry the mutation. There may, therefore, be a clump of egg cells that carry the mutation, though the majority of her eggs will not. This is known as germline mosaicism.

MIGHT THE BROTHERS OF THE AFFECTED BOY ALSO BE AFFECTED?

If the condition is not obvious at birth but presents in childhood (e.g. Duchenne muscular dystrophy), and other male infants have been born subsequent to the affected boy, it is possible that they also carry the gene mutation. This will obviously cause major concerns for the parents, who may wish to have these younger sons tested. The issue of testing children has been discussed in previous chapters (4 & 8). In this situation, testing will be offered. It will clarify the situation for the parents and, if the child is found to carry the mutation, allow for referral to the appropriate paediatrician before symptoms of the condition present. It might also be an influential factor in the parents' decisions about family planning.

ARE THE SISTERS OF THE AFFECTED BOY LIKELY TO BE CARRIERS?

If the mother is a carrier then each of her daughters will have a 1 in 2 (50%) risk of being a carrier. If the mother was not shown to be a carrier but has a residual risk of germline mosaicism then her daughters will have a very low risk of being a carrier. Carrier tests are not offered to such females during childhood as their carrier status will only be significant when planning a family. The parents will be advised that testing will be offered to their daughter when she is about 16 years old (or sooner if she is anxious to know or becomes sexually active). It is common practice to write to the GP informing them of the girl's risk of being a carrier so that there is a record in her medical notes.

ARE THERE ANY PRENATAL TESTS AVAILABLE FOR FUTURE PREGNANCIES?

The answer to this question will always be yes, but the type of test and amount of information available will depend on whether the gene alteration is detectable and, if not, whether family studies will be informative. Ideally, these factors need to be determined and discussed with the couple before a subsequent pregnancy occurs.

If the gene mutation is detectable, prenatal diagnosis using CVS or amniocentesis (see Chapter 5) will be available. The laboratory will be able to report the sex of the foetus within 48 hours. If the foetus is male, further tests will determine whether the gene mutation is present.

If the gene mutation is not detectable, it may be possible to determine which of the maternal X chromosomes carries the altered gene by the use of family linkage studies.

Linkage Studies

Imagine that the location of the gene for the disorder is known but the gene cannot yet be 'read'. It is, however, known that immediately after the gene there are a number of repeats of the triplet DNA bases ACG. The number of times ACG is repeated is irrelevant because this is junk DNA, but these repeats may be useful in differentiating between the X chromosomes in a family. These repeats are referred to as 'markers'. Let us consider how this may help the family in Pedigree 9.1.

Blood is obtained from Sarah and the results show that it will be possible to differentiate between her two X chromosomes:

1. (*gene that cannot be 'read'*) ACG ACG ACG; and
2. (*gene that cannot be 'read'*) ACG ACG ACG ACG ACG ACG.

The X chromosome with three repeats is labelled 'A' and the X chromosome with six repeats is labelled 'B'.

Blood is obtained from the two affected males, Jake and Paul, and from both of Sarah's parents and her unaffected brother, David. The results of all these tests are shown in Pedigree 9.4.

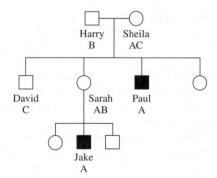

Pedigree 9.4

- Sarah's X chromosomes are patterned A and B.
- Her brother, Paul, and son, Jake, both affected, carry pattern A (remember that as males they only have one copy of the X chromosome).
- Her mother, Sheila (whom we know must also be a carrier as she has an affected son and a carrier daughter), has patterns A and C.
- It would therefore appear that the altered gene is carried on the X chromosome with pattern A:

    1. Sarah has inherited her X chromosome with pattern B from her father.
    2. David has inherited the X chromosome with pattern C from his mother.

The results in this family are informative. However, because the tests do not look directly at the gene alteration they are not 100% accurate. Molecular geneticists will be able to estimate how accurate the results are and linkage studies with accuracy of less than 95% will not be used (For some conditions the 'marker' may be within the gene when the results of the linkage study will be highly accurate.) These studies are time consuming and should preferably be carried out before a pregnancy. Not all studies will be informative as there may be no clear distinctions in patterns. If Sarah's father had pattern A and both Sarah's X chromosomes showed the pattern A, linkage studies would not have been possible in this family.

If the results of a linkage study are informative, it is important to discuss their limitations with the couple. 95% accuracy means that if a test suggests that a male foetus carries the high-risk X chromosome, there is a 5% chance that it is unaffected. Conversely, if the test suggests that the male foetus carries the low-risk X chromosome then there is a 5% risk that it is affected.

The possibility for prenatal testing will depend on the outcome of the linkage study. If the study was informative, prenatal testing will be possible. The sex of the foetus will be known within 48 hours and, if male, the linkage study will determine if the high-risk X chromosome has been inherited.

If the linkage study was uninformative then the only prenatal test available will be foetal sexing, with a view to terminating any male foetus. This raises several difficult issues, depending on whether the woman knows her carrier status.

If the woman knows she is a carrier, the couple knows that each time they terminate a male foetus there is a 1 in 2 (50%) risk that it was unaffected.

If she does not know her carrier status, the couple will know that there is a possibility that she is not a carrier and that each time a pregnancy with a male foetus is terminated, it may well have been unaffected. They should also consider that within the woman's lifetime it may become possible to determine her carrier status. If this were to show that she was a carrier, they would know that each male foetus terminated had a 1 in 2 possibility of being unaffected; if it were to show that she was not a carrier, they would know that all the male foetuses terminated had been unaffected.

Couples have to make these decisions with the information that is available within their reproductive lifespan. The severity of the disorder and the effect of an affected male relative on their lives may have a strong influence on their decisions (see Case Study 3).

CAN FEMALE CARRIERS OF THE ALTERED GENE BE AFFECTED?

As a general rule, females who carry an altered copy of a gene on the X chromosome will not be affected as they also carry a normal copy of that gene. Only one copy of each gene on the X chromosome is necessary in both males and females to produce the required amount of gene product. However, because of this there is a mechanism in females known as X inactivation, which prevents them from having too much gene product. This occurs early in embryonic life, when one copy of the X chromosome in each cell in the female embryo is made inactive, or switched off. This usually happens randomly, with an equal proportion of the paternally derived and maternally derived X chromosomes being inactivated. Non-random or skewed inactivation may occur, in which case more copies of either the paternally derived X chromosome or the maternally derived X chromosome are inactivated. If this happens when a gene alteration has been inherited from one parent, it may result in a female carrier being affected with an X-linked recessive condition since many of her normal copies of the gene have been inactivated. The affected female will usually have milder symptoms than an affected male as she will still have some active X chromosomes carrying the normal copy of the gene.

CASE STUDY 1: DUCHENNE MUSCULAR DYSTROPHY

Harry was referred to a paediatrician by his GP when he was 2 1/2 years old. Harry had two older sisters and a younger brother. His mother, Jeanette, was concerned because he had difficulty running, was unable to ride a bike and tended to climb up stairs on all fours. She had also noticed that he was later than his sisters to start walking, at around 20 months. She thought he might have weak ankles and need support boots. The paediatrician, however, suspected a much more serious diagnosis: Duchenne muscular dystrophy.

DUCHENNE MUSCULAR DYSTROPHY: THE DISEASE

Duchenne muscular dystrophy (DMD) is inherited as an X-linked condition. It is characterised by progressive muscle weakness. The early signs already noted by Harry's mother are typical of the condition as the first muscles to be affected are the strong thigh muscles. The paediatrician noticed that Harry's thigh muscles looked thin, while his calf muscles were overdeveloped for a child of his age. The muscle weakness progresses over a period of years, with most boys being confined to a wheelchair by their early teens. Gradually the muscles of the upper body become affected and eventually the respiratory muscles are involved. Death usually occurs in the late teens or early twenties.

The clinical diagnosis may be confirmed by blood tests:

1. DNA analysis. In 65% of affected boys a large deletion is found in the gene. In a further 30% of boys a point mutation (i.e. only one DNA base is altered) is found and in the remaining 5% a duplication of DNA material is found.
2. Creatinine kinase (CK) levels. This is an enzyme produced by muscles during exercise. The normal levels range between 24 and 170 u/l. In an affected boy, the levels will be 1000 u/l or above.

The paediatrician explained his suspicions and took blood to confirm the diagnosis. Jeanette and her husband, Roy, were devastated. They had expected to be told that Harry had a minor condition and instead were told that he had a terminal illness. The couple was seen again when the results of the tests were available and these confirmed the diagnosis. The paediatrician suggested referral to the local clinical genetics service to discuss the possible implications for future pregnancies and other family members, and the couple readily agreed to this.

GENETIC COUNSELLING

Initially the couple was seen by the genetic counsellor in a family history clinic. The purpose of this consultation was to obtain a detailed family history, which in this case showed that no other males in the previous three generations had been affected. This raised the question of whether the gene alteration occurred as a new mutation in Harry or Jeanette, or whether it had been present in previous generations without resulting in the birth of an affected male. The consultation was also important in allowing Jeanette and Roy an opportunity to explore their feelings about the diagnosis and its impact on the family.

DETECTING THE SOURCE OF THE GENE MUTATION

Jeanette was very tearful when talking about Harry and had strong feelings of guilt about the thought that she might have passed an altered gene to her son. The

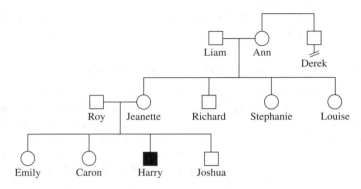

Pedigree 9.5

GC used diagrams to demonstrate X-linked recessive inheritance to the couple and explained that the gene alteration may have occurred for the first time in Harry. Jeanette needed reassurance that there was nothing in the family history that could have forewarned her that she might be a carrier for DMD. As the gene deletion had been found in Harry, blood tests would be able to determine Jeanette's carrier status, and she was keen for these tests to be carried out. Blood was therefore taken from Jeanette for DNA analysis and to determine CK levels. CK levels in carrier women will be elevated above normal, but not to the same extent as in an affected male. A second sample of blood needed to be taken a week later for repeat CK level testing, as there can be variations according to the amount of activity prior to venepuncture. The GC arranged this second test via the GP and advised Jeanette not to undergo any strenuous exercise in the 24 hours prior to her next blood test. A clinic appointment was arranged for three weeks' time, when the results would be available.

The results of Jeanette's tests showed that she was a carrier as she had the same gene deletion found in Harry. The impact of being a carrier for an X-linked recessive condition may be much greater than that for being a carrier of an autosomal recessive condition. In the latter case, both parents have to pass on the altered gene for the child to be affected (Chapter 8). With an X-linked condition, only the mother passes on the altered gene, while herself remaining unaffected. Support needs to be given to allow the mother to come to terms with her carrier status.

Confirmation that Jeanette was a carrier for DMD also had implications for the extended family.

IMPLICATIONS FOR THE AFFECTED BOY'S SIBLINGS

The couple wanted to know if their other son was affected. Joshua had a 1 in 2 (50%) risk of having inherited the gene deletion. Although genetic testing of children for carrier status or adult onset disorders is not usually offered (Chapter 5), in this situation the disorder occurs in early childhood. A blood test was therefore arranged for Joshua and, to his parents' great relief, this showed that he had inherited the normal copy of the gene from his mother.

Jeanette and Roy were also concerned about the gene status of their daughters, Emily, aged 7, and Caron, aged 5. Both girls were at a 1 in 2 (50%) risk of being a carrier, but knowing their gene status would not affect their management and therefore carrier testing was not offered. With their parents' consent, a letter about each girl was sent to her GP, advising that they be referred for genetic counselling when around 16 years of age, or sooner if there were concerns about possible pregnancy.

Although the couple was not planning to extend their family, Jeanette needed to know if prenatal testing would be available if she became pregnant again. She was assured that prenatal diagnosis would be available in any future pregnancy.

CARRIER TESTING THE EXTENDED FAMILY

Jeanette's mother and sisters were concerned to know if they were carriers. Jeanette's mother, Ann, was tested first and her results showed that she did not carry the gene deletion. There was therefore only a small residual risk that her other daughters, Stephanie and Louise, were carriers, if Ann had germline mosaicism. No other members of the family were at risk of being carriers. Stephanie and Louise requested carrier testing as they were both very worried about any potential risk of having an affected son. The results of their tests showed that neither of them carried the gene deletion.

CASE STUDY 2: FRAGILE X SYNDROME

Simon's parents, Lucy and Jamie, first became concerned about their son when he was two years old. Compared with his cousins of a similar age he was slow to speak, and he seemed to have poor co-ordination. Their GP referred Simon to a paediatrician, who agreed with the parents' concerns and noted that Simon was slightly delayed in his motor development. The paediatrician explained to the parents that he was concerned Simon was displaying signs of a developmental delay in several areas and that the most likely cause was a genetic condition, which could be detected by a blood test.

Several weeks later the results of the test confirmed that Simon had Fragile X syndrome. Lucy and Jamie were horrified when the diagnosis and its prognosis were explained as they were both high achievers with university degrees and had never considered that their children might not be as bright as they were. They were even more devastated at receiving the news at this time as Lucy had just had a positive pregnancy test. An urgent appointment with the genetic counselling service was requested and the couple was seen within 48 hours.

FRAGILE X SYNDROME: THE DISORDER

Fragile X is the second most common cause of mental retardation in boys (the most common being Down syndrome), and the most common inherited cause. Although it is inherited as an X-linked recessive condition occurring mainly in boys, girls can also be affected, but less commonly and usually less severely.

Boys with Fragile X have learning difficulties ranging from mild to severe. They may have delayed speech and language development, behavioural problems and some features of autism. Physical features include a relatively large head with a long face, prominent ears and large jaw and, following puberty, large testes.

Girls with the Fragile X gene mutation may have normal intelligence but about half of them will have mild to moderate learning and behavioural problems similar to, but less severe than, those experienced by affected males. 'However, more subtle problems with learning, behavioural, and emotional difficulties are common even in females with a full mutation who have a normal IQ' (Firth & Hurst, 2005, p. 324).

THE FRAGILE X GENE

At the beginning of the Fragile X gene (called FMR1), a small part (CGG) is repeated a variable number of times. For individuals with Fragile X syndrome the number of repeats is much larger than normal. This is known as an expansion. The size of the expansion varies between individuals.

- People with up to 55 repeats have a normal copy of the gene.
- People with 55–200 repeats are carriers of what is known as a premutation and are unaffected. Females who carry the premutation can pass it on unchanged, but it may expand into a full mutation. Males who carry the premutation will always pass it on as a premutation. Both male and female carriers of premutations were once considered to be clinically uninvolved. However, it is now known that premutation males can develop a Fragile X associated tremor/ataxia (FXTAS) over the age of 50. Females with premutations are at an increased risk for premature ovarian failure (POF) (McConkie-Rosell et al., 2005).
- People with over 200 repeats have a full mutation. When this occurs the gene is switched off and doesn't function properly, causing Fragile X syndrome.

GENETIC COUNSELLING

Lucy and Jamie were stunned by the diagnosis in their son. Lucy was now six weeks pregnant and anxious to know how quickly she could find out about the risk to this pregnancy. A detailed family history showed that Simon was the only person in the family known to have developmental delay, although he had several cousins who were still only a few months old.

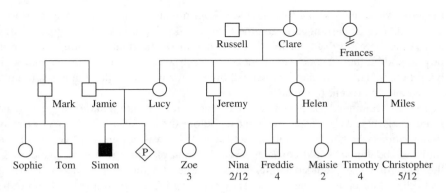

Pedigree 9.6

RISK TO CURRENT PREGNANCY

This would depend on whether there was an expansion in the FMR1 gene on either of Lucy's X chromosomes.

- If Lucy had the normal number of repeats at the beginning of the gene (i.e. up to 55) then the mutation might have occurred for the first time in Simon, although there would be a residual risk of germline mosaicism.
- If Lucy carried the premutation (i.e. 55–200 repeats) then each of her children would have a 1 in 2 (50%) risk of inheriting it from her. If the size of the mutation remained unchanged, they would be carriers. If it expanded to a full mutation, boys would definitely be affected and girls might be.
- If Lucy carried a full mutation (i.e. over 200 repeats) then each of her children would have a 1 in 2 (50%) risk of inheriting it from her. Again, any boys who inherited it would definitely be affected and any girls who inherited it might be.

The results of Lucy's test showed that she carried the premutation. The couple therefore requested prenatal diagnosis and opted for CVS at 11 weeks' gestation. The test procedure, together with associated risks, was explained in detail (see Chapter 5).

The couple was told that the sex of the baby would be known within 48 hours:

- If it was male, further tests would determine whether he had inherited an expanded copy of the gene.
- If it was a female, further tests would only be carried out if the couple wished to terminate a female with the full mutation, even though she might be unaffected or only mildly affected.

Lucy and Jamie both felt that they would only want to continue with this pregnancy if the baby did not carry the full mutation. Sadly, the results of the CVS showed that the baby was a male with a full mutation. A termination of pregnancy was therefore arranged. The GC arranged to see the couple following this to give support. Lucy and Jamie were very sad but felt that they had made the right decision. Simon was now attending the child development centre each week and they were pleased with his progress. They felt that they needed time to recover from the diagnoses in both Simon and the recent pregnancy.

The GC reminded Lucy that women who carry the premutation appear to be more likely to have an early menopause, before the age of 40. There was no way to determine whether this would affect Lucy. Lucy was currently 28 years old and said she and Jamie would consider this fact when planning future pregnancies. In the meantime, the extended family was concerned for the couple but also worried that other children might be at risk. They had asked Lucy to arrange for them to be seen by the GC.

TESTING THE EXTENDED FAMILY

The GC arranged an appointment to see Lucy's parents, Russell and Clare. They too had been devastated by Simon's diagnosis and found it difficult to accept as they had thought he was just 'a bit lazy' and would soon be speaking well and doing everything else that children of his age did. They were also worried that tests might show that one of them carried the gene expansion but felt that it was important for them to be tested so that more information was available to their other children. X-linked recessive inheritance was explained and then there was a discussion of who else in the family might be at risk. They realised that their younger daughter, Helen, might be a carrier. They also realised that as their sons were unaffected they could not have inherited the full mutation. However, if Clare had a premutation then her sons might have inherited this and could pass it on to their daughters. Russell had no siblings and Clare's only sister was now aged 59 years and had no children.

The couple felt that now the question of their gene status had been raised they would like to pursue testing whatever the outcome. Blood samples were obtained from both of them and it was agreed that the GC would phone with the results. These showed that Russell carried the premutation and Clare had two normal copies of the gene. Russell was very upset by this news but glad that the situation had been clarified for Helen. He realised that she must have inherited his premutation and that there was a potential risk to her children.

However, at the age of four her first son, Freddie, had an extensive vocabulary and could already read and write some basic words so there were no concerns about his development. Maisie, just two years old, was already a chatterbox, and at her recent development assessment was noted to be very advanced in her verbal skills. There was a 1 in 2 (50%) possibility that Maisie was a carrier of the premutation, and her parents agreed to contact the genetics service again when she was about 16 years old. Maisie's father, Peter, had had a vasectomy a year earlier so he and Helen did not expect to have any further additions to their family. Helen was aware that if she were to contemplate further pregnancies in the future, either by AID or with a new partner, there would be a risk, but she felt that both those scenarios were highly unlikely to occur.

CASE STUDY 3: MENTAL RETARDATION OF UNKNOWN AETIOLOGY

When Mark and Jane decided to start a family they asked their GP to refer them for genetic counselling because of Jane's strong family history of mental retardation and behavioural problems. Jane had two brothers and a nephew who were affected and she was aware that there were other affected relatives in the extended family. She had no clear idea of how many, but thought they were all males. The couple was also concerned because Jane was 36 years old.

GENETIC COUNSELLING

When Jane saw the genetic counsellor at the family history clinic she brought her mother, Mary, with her so that an accurate family history could be obtained. All the affected individuals in the family were male and all showed signs of delay in childhood, with the degree of severity ranging from moderate to severe.

IMPACT OF THE DISORDER ON THE FAMILY

Jane's uncle, James, was severely affected and had been in residential care since his teenage years. Jane's brothers, Robert and Timothy, both lived at home but attended a day centre and had weekend respite care once a month to give Jane's parents a break. Jane and her other siblings worried about who would care for their brothers when their parents died or became unable to manage.

Jane was only too aware of the effect of having several mentally retarded children within the nuclear family. Jane felt that her childhood had been detrimentally affected by having two mentally retarded brothers. She had had less attention from her parents than she should have because so much of their time was taken up with looking after Robert and Timothy and dealing with their challenging behaviour. Family outings and holidays often became nightmares of embarrassment for her due to her brothers' behaviour. She had been unable to bring friends home to play as they were often scared of her brothers and because her brothers interrupted all activities.

Jane was also very aware of the impact of her brothers on her parents' marriage. Although her parents' relationship was strong and had survived, it had been adversely affected by the strain of looking after two affected children. They had always been stressed and tired, as the boys' sleeping patterns were erratic, and they had seldom been able to have time by themselves as finding babysitters was a problem. As Jane's parents got older and lost the stamina to cope, the problems

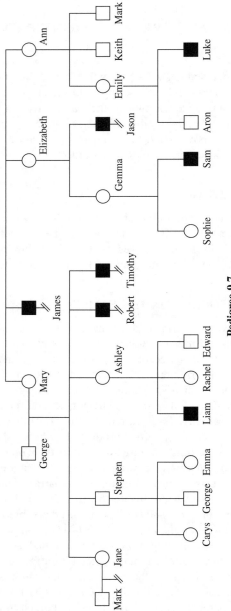

Pedigree 9.7

increased. There was also the question of what would happen to the boys when their parents died.

CLARIFYING THE DIAGNOSIS

As far as the family was aware, no cause for the mental retardation and behavioural problems had ever been found. Permission was given to obtain the hospital notes for Robert and Timothy, and for Jane's nephew, Liam, and when all the relevant information had been obtained an appointment was made for Mark and Jane to attend the genetic clinic.

The geneticist explained that no obvious cause had been found to account for the mental retardation and behavioural problems. Chromosome studies had proved normal and Fragile X syndrome had been excluded. No unusual physical characteristics had been found in Robert, Timothy or Liam to suggest a different syndrome.

The pattern of affected males in the family suggested that it was an X-linked recessive condition. The pedigree indicated that Mary, Ashley, Elizabeth, Gemma, Ann and Emily were carriers. Although Ann had had two unaffected sons, her daughter, Emily, had an affected boy. Jane therefore had a 1 in 2 (50%) risk of being a carrier and a 1 in 8 ((1 in 2) X (1 in 4)) risk of having an affected son.

PRENATAL DIAGNOSTIC OPTIONS

As there was no definitive diagnosis in the affected males, there was no definitive prenatal test available. The geneticist explained that it might be possible to trace the high-risk X chromosome within the family, and the couple was keen to pursue this. Over the next few weeks, blood samples were obtained from Mary, Robert, Timothy and Ashley, and the family was made aware that the results might take some time.

Unfortunately, none of the markers used by the laboratory proved to be informative and when Mark and Jane were seen again they were told that the only prenatal test available to them at that time was foetal sexing. Mark and Jane had considered this outcome while waiting for the results of the family linkage studies and had decided that if it proved to be the case they would opt for foetal sexing, with a view to terminating male foetuses. They had come to this decision after much heart searching. Jane felt that she had missed out on a normal childhood, and had avoided serious relationships for a long time in her early adult life. Now that she was happily married she did not want her relationship with Mark to be strained by the burden of an affected child. But nor did she want to miss out on the opportunity to have children.

The couple was aware that they might terminate an unaffected male. They were also aware that there was a possibility that any daughters they might have would be carriers, but hoped that by the time those daughters had reached childbearing age, more tests would be available.

Jane told the geneticist that while waiting for the results of the linkage studies she had discovered that she was already pregnant, and was currently at nine weeks' gestation. The couple requested an early prenatal test to exclude Down syndrome and to determine the sex of the baby, and CVS was arranged. On this occasion the results showed a female infant with 46 chromosomes. Mark and Jane were delighted not to have been faced with the decision to terminate but were aware that it might still be a possibility if they decided to extend their family in the future.

OTHER SEX-LINKED CONDITIONS

X-LINKED DOMINANT

These conditions are much less common but some examples are:

- Vitamin D-resistant rickets.
- X-linked dominant retinitis pigmentosa.
- Incontinentia pigmentosa.
- Rett's syndrome.

Both males and females can be affected with this form of inheritance. Females may be less severely affected because X inactivation means that they have two types of X chromosome, one with the normal copy of the gene and one with the altered gene. Males are assumed to be more severely affected, and some conditions may be incompatible with normal male foetal development. In those conditions where males do not survive a pregnancy there will be an excess number of females born into the family.

Each child of an affected female will have a 1 in 2 (50%) risk of being affected. All male offspring of affected males will be unaffected, as they inherit their father's Y chromosome, but all female offspring of affected males will be affected. The pattern shown in the pedigree below may initially be mistaken for autosomal dominant inheritance, but there will be no male to male transmission.

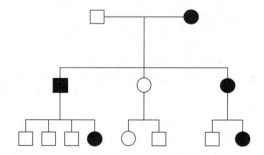

Figure 9.3 A Typical X-Linked Dominant Pedigree.

Y-LINKED INHERITANCE

This form of inheritance is even less common. Only males will be affected and all their sons will inherit the condition. Their daughters will inherit their normal X chromosome and will neither be affected nor carriers for the condition. Recent evidence suggests that some forms of male infertility are caused by gene mutations on the Y chromosome (Mueller & Young, 2001, p. 105). If affected men are helped to reproduce by technologies such as intracytoplasmic sperm injection (ICSI) then any male offspring so produced may also be sub-fertile (Mueller & Young, 2001, p. 105).

POINTS FOR REFLECTION

- How might you feel about yourself if you knew you might pass on a disorder to your sons?
- How do you feel about the termination of male foetuses that are not known to be definitely affected?
- How might your feelings influence the way you deal with prospective parents?

REFERENCES

Firth, H.V. and Hurst, J.A. (2005) *Oxford Desk Reference: Clinical Genetics*, Oxford University Press, Oxford.

McConkie-Rosell, A. *et al.* (2005) Genetic counseling for Fragile X syndrome: Updated recommendations of the National Society of Genetic Counselors. *Journal of Genetic Counseling*, 4(14), 249–70.

Mueller, R.F. and Young, I.D. (2001) *Emery's Elements of Medical Genetics*, 11th edn, Churchill Livingstone, London.

10 Multifactorial Inheritance: Interaction of Genes and Environment

JO HAYDON

If a male inherits a gene mutation for Duchenne muscular dystrophy, he will develop that condition regardless of the environment in which he is brought up. If an individual has no dietary intake of vitamin C over a prolonged period, it won't matter how genetically 'fit' that individual is, they will develop scurvy. These are examples of disorders caused solely by genetic or environmental factors. However, there are many common diseases and malformations that show a familial tendency but, within a family, do not occur as frequently as single gene disorders. These are referred to as multifactorial conditions and it is thought that their inheritance is controlled by many genes, each with a small additive effect, as well as by the effect of the environment. The number of genes involved can be variable and some will play a more important role than others, but no one gene is dominant over or recessive to another. Typically, only one organ system is affected. A combination of genetic and environmental factors contribute to many of our normal characteristics and it may be useful to consider these first before looking at multifactorial disorders.

Most normal human characteristics are determined as continuous multifactorial traits. That is, they have a continuously variable distribution within the population. Common examples of these characteristics are blood pressure, head circumference, height and intelligence quotient.

If height were determined by two equally frequent alleles (alternative forms of a gene found at the same location on an individual chromosome pair), a 'tall' and a 'short' allele, this would result in three possible heights in a ratio of 1:2:1 (see Table 10.1).

If height were determined by four equally frequent alleles found on two pairs of genes, this would result in five heights in a ratio of 1:4:6:4:1 (see Table 10.2). That is:

1: 4 tall alleles
4: 3 tall and 1 short alleles
6: 2 tall and 2 short alleles
4: 1 tall and 3 short alleles
1: 4 short alleles.

Genetics in Practice: A clinical approach for healthcare practitioners Edited by Jo Haydon
© 2007 John Wiley & Sons, Ltd

Table 10.1 Height Determined by Two Alleles

Parent 1's
alleles

	a	b	
a	aa (tall)	ab (medium)	**Key** a: allele for tall height b: allele for short height
b	ab (medium)	bb (short)	

Parent 2's
alleles

offspring

Table 10.2 Height Determined by Four Alleles

Parent 1's
alleles

	ac	ad	bc	bd
ac	aacc (4 tall)	aacd (3 tall, 1 short)	abcc (3 tall, 1 short)	abcd (2 tall, 2 short)
ad	aacd (3 tall, 1 short)	aadd (2 tall, 2 short)	abcd (2 tall, 2 short)	abdd (1 tall, 3 short)
bc	abcc (3 tall, 1 short)	abcd (2 tall, 2 short)	bbcc (2 tall, 2 short)	bbcd (1 tall, 3 short)
bd	abcd (2 tall, 2 short)	abdd (1 tall, 3 short)	bbcd (1 tall, 3 short)	bbdd (4 short)

Parent 2's
alleles

offspring

Key
a: allele for tall height
b: allele for short height
c: allele for tall height
d: allele for short height

If height were determined by six equally frequent alleles found on three pairs of genes, this would result in seven heights in a ratio of 1:6:15:21:15:6:1 (see Figure 10.1). You may wish to draw up a table similar to Table 10.2 with the eight combinations of parental alleles that would result, i.e. ace, acf, ade, adf, bce, bcf, bde, bdf. You should find the following combinations:

1: 6 tall alleles
6: 5 tall and 1 short alleles
15: 4 tall and 2 short alleles
21: 3 tall and 3 short alleles
15: 2 tall and 4 short alleles
6: 1 tall and 5 short alleles
1: 6 short alleles.

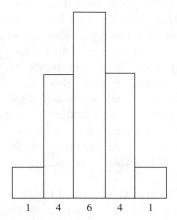

1   4   6   4   1

Figure 10.1 Diagram Showing Shape of Height Distribution when Four Alleles are Involved

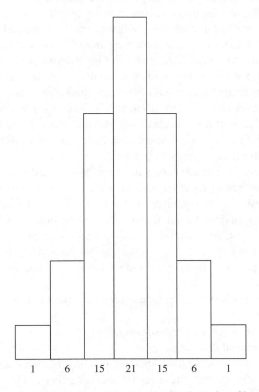

1   6   15   21   15   6   1

Figure 10.2 Diagram Showing Shape of Height Distribution when Six Alleles are Involved

These characteristics show a continuous distribution within the general population, known as a normal distribution. This distribution can be generated by the action of many genes at different locations, with each one exerting an equal additive effect. This is represented in a symmetrical bell-shaped curve distributed evenly around a mean (the mean height is the sum of the height of all the individuals measured, divided by the number of those individuals).

At the lower end of the curve would be an individual with six short alleles, and at the higher end, an individual with six tall alleles. Environmental factors also play a part. Chronic malnutrition or starvation in childhood would limit the growth of an individual to less than their genetic potential for height. However, individuals with six short alleles would be liable to be short whatever their dietary intake in childhood.

The liability of a population to be tall would follow a normal distribution curve, with most people showing moderate height. Only when a certain threshold of liability is exceeded would an individual be tall. In this case the threshold may be reached when an individual has five or six tall genes. Relatives of a tall person would have a greater liability to be taller than the general population as they would be more likely to have inherited a higher number of tall genes.

Family studies, particularly those including twins, have helped to determine how important genetic factors are in determining human characteristics. Monozygotic twins are genetically identical, share the same intrauterine environment and, unless separated at birth, are raised in a common environment. Dizygotic twins are only on average 50% genetically identical, but share the same intrauterine environment and, unless separated at birth, are raised in a common environment. Siblings are on average 50% genetically identical but do not share a common intrauterine environment. Their family environment also differs as they are never at the same age when an environmental factor is present.

Comparisons have been made between monozygotic and dizygotic twins, between monozygotic twins raised together and separated at birth and between dizygotic twins raised together and separated at birth, to try to determine how important genetic versus environmental factors are. When both members of a pair of twins exhibit the same trait, they are said to be concordant. Studies (Connor & Ferguson-Smith, 1984, p. 92) have looked at height and IQ in twins who were divided into two groups – monozygotic and dizygotic – and the following results were found:

For both these traits, genetic factors are very important but environmental factors also play a part.

Similar studies (Connor & Ferguson-Smith, 1984, p. 93) have been used when looking at multifactorial disorders:

Although with each disease the incidence of concordance is higher in monozygotic than dizygotic twins, the importance of genetic factors is very variable, ranging from 70% in manic depressive psychology to only 19% in heart disease.

Table 10.3 Concordance between Monozygotic and Dizygotic Twins for Height and IQ

Trait	Monozygotic %	Dizygotic %
Height	95	52
IQ	90	60

Table 10.4 Concordance between Monozygotic and Dizygotic Twins for Various Multifactorial Disorders

Disease	Monozygotic twins %	Dizygotic twins %
Manic depression	70	15
Schizophrenia	45	12
Epilepsy	37	10
Cleft lip and palate	35	5
Ischaemic heart disease	19	8

By use of these studies, it has been possible to estimate the heritability of various disorders. Heritability is the proportion of the cause owing to genetic rather than environmental factors.

COMMON MULTIFACTORIAL CONDITIONS

- Congenital malformations:

  1. cleft lip/palate
  2. congenital dislocation of the hip
  3. congenital heart defects
  4. neural tube defects
  5. pyloric stenosis
  6. talipes.

- Later onset disorders:

  1. asthma
  2. diabetes mellitus
  3. epilepsy
  4. glaucoma
  5. hypertension
  6. ischaemic heart disease
  7. schizophrenia
  8. manic depression.

EMPIRIC RISKS

These are estimates based on observation and experience, rather than calculations based on the mechanism by which the condition is inherited. These risks are based on population studies looking at the frequency of particular disorders in given populations. Data collected on one population may not apply to other populations (Harper, 2004, p. 57), e.g. the incidence and recurrence rates of neural tube defects are very different between a Japanese population and a Northern Irish population. It is therefore vital to ensure that the data you are looking at applies to a similar population to that of your patient. You must also take into account the severity of the disease and number of affected relatives, as these can further affect the risk to the patient.

Multifactorial inheritance is likely if:

- The condition is relatively common.
- The incidence in relatives is lower than would be expected for Mendelian inheritance but higher than that in the general population.
- The incidence is greatest amongst relatives of the most severely affected individuals, e.g. the recurrence risk for bilateral cleft lip and palate is 6%, but for unilateral cleft lip and palate is 2%. It is thought that the more severely affected individual has more detrimental genes than the mildly affected individual.
- The recurrence risk is greater if more than one close relative is affected.
- The recurrence risk to siblings is the same as the risk to offspring.
- The recurrence risk decreases rapidly the more distant the relative.
- The recurrence risk is higher when the index case is of the least commonly affected sex.

There are a number of multifactorial conditions with an unequal sex ratio (see Table 10.5; Connor & Ferguson-Smith, 1984, p. 96).

Pyloric stenosis affects 5 in 1000 males but only 1 in 1000 females, which means that the threshold for affect is higher for females than males (Connor & Ferguson-Smith, 1984, p. 96). Therefore, if a female presents with pyloric stenosis it is likely that the genetic factors involved are greater than in an affected male. The increase above population risk for relatives of the affected female will be greater than the increase above population risk for relatives of an affected male. However, because

Table 10.5 Sex Ratio (Male to Female) for Various Multifactorial Disorders

Disorder	Ratio male to female
Pyloric stenosis	5 to 1
Hirschprung disease	3 to 1
Congenital dislocation of hip	1 to 6
Talipes	2 to 1

Table 10.6 Increased Risk According to Sex of Affected Individual

Relationship	Population risk%	Increase on general population risk	Actual risk%
female relative of female patient	1/70	X 70	1
male relative of female patient	1/2	X 35	17
male relative of male patient	1	X 5	5
female relative of male patient	1	X 2	2

the incidence of pyloric stenosis is higher in males, the actual risk to sons will be greater than the risk to daughters, as illustrated in Table 10.6.

Multifactorial inheritance is more complex than single gene inheritance and it may be more difficult to give precise recurrence risks in each situation. Also, although a number of genes are thought to be involved, it is not yet possible to test for these genes to determine which individuals within a family are more at risk. With some conditions the environmental factors involved are well recognised and it is therefore possible for individuals to modify their behaviour in order to minimise their risk.

CASE STUDY 1: CONGENITAL ABNORMALITY

When Jeanette was pregnant for the second time she eagerly awaited her routine detailed scan at 20 weeks' gestation. She remembered how excited she and her husband Mark had been when she first saw her son Ethan, now aged 3 years, on the ultrasound scan. However, on this occasion their excitement led to dismay when they were told that there may be a problem. A senior sonographer rescanned the baby and told Jeanette that the baby's spine had not formed properly and the baby had the condition known as spina bifida.

NEURAL TUBE DEFECT: THE CONDITION

A neural tube defect (NTD) is a failure of complete closure of the neural tube during early embryonic life. The incidence varies according to geographical location and a high proportion of affected foetuses abort spontaneously. The degree of severity is variable and there are three main types of defect:

1. **Anencephaly**, in which there is complete absence of the vault of the skull. This is not compatible with survival for more than a few hours. The majority of cases will be diagnosed in the antenatal period due to raised maternal serum alpha-feta protein and ultrasound scan appearance.

2. **Encephalocele**, in which the meninges herniate through the skull bones and may also contain brain tissue.
3. **Spina bifida**, in which the defect occurs at the lower end of the neural tube, leading to a myelomeningocele (open lesion) or meningocele (skin covered sac). Large lumbar-sacral lesions usually cause paralysis of the lower limbs and impaired bladder and bowel function. A milder form, spinal bifida occulta, is a closed defect of the bony arch which rarely causes any problems.

When a neural tube defect occurs, it is most likely to be an isolated malformation, but it may be due to chromosomal abnormality, e.g. trisomy 13 and trisomy 18, or a single gene abnormality, such as Meckel's syndrome, inherited as an autosomal recessive disorder.

If it occurs as an isolated malformation, it is thought to be multifactorial.

Genetic factors include:

• A mutation in the folate receptor gene, causing interference with folic acid absorption.
• Being of Celtic origin.

Environmental factors include:

• Poor socioeconomic state.
• Multiparity.
• Folic acid embryopathy; this latter may be due to poor folic acid intake or interference with absorption caused by anti-convulsant therapy or insulin-dependent diabetes.

The findings on ultrasound indicated a severe form of the condition and the couple decided to terminate the pregnancy. It was a decision taken with great sadness, but Jeanette and Mark felt that the baby's quality of life would be poor and they also worried about the effect that a severely disabled child would have on other family members, especially Ethan.

When Jeanette attended her follow-up appointment, her main questions related to why the condition had occurred and what the risk of recurrence was. Often this information is given by the obstetrician, but Jeanette also had lots of questions about the extended family and she was therefore referred to the clinical genetics service.

GENETIC COUNSELLING

Jeanette and Mark were seen by a genetic counsellor two months after the termination had taken place. They were still feeling very sad and guilty that they had decided to end the pregnancy. The GC spent some time exploring these issues with the couple and then obtained a detailed family history. As expected, there had been no previous individuals in the family with a neural tube defect.

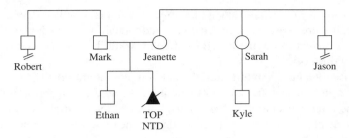

Pedigree 10.1

The GC explained that NTD is thought to be caused by a combination of genetic and environmental factors. Once it has occurred, the risk of recurrence for a couple is around 3% (depending on the geographical incidence) (Harper, 2004, p. 187). One of the environmental factors is poor absorption of folic acid and the GC told Jeanette that the 3% risk could be reduced to 1% if she were to take folic acid 5 mg for three months prior to conception and during the early weeks of pregnancy. Jeanette became very upset at this point, thinking that it was her fault that her folic acid levels may not have been sufficient. The GC explained that the information given about Jeanette's diet indicated that it was adequate, and told her that in some individuals the folate receptor gene does not function properly and an adequate dietary intake is not sufficient to ensure adequate absorption. Jeanette was advised to see her GP for a prescription for folic acid 5 mg daily (the dosage of tablets that can be bought without prescription is only 0.4 mg).

Jeanette wanted to know if there were any early diagnostic tests available as she had found terminating the pregnancy at 20 weeks' gestation very distressing. She had already felt the baby moving and many people had been aware of the pregnancy. Her family and friends had been very supportive of her decision to terminate but she had found it difficult to tell them. Although the results of a MSAFP (maternal serum alpha-foeto protein) screening test may indicate that a foetus is at an increased risk of NTD, the definitive diagnosis can only be made on USS or amniocentesis. The GC explained that an earlier scan of 12 weeks' gestation would detect the most severe form, i.e. anencephaly, but that spina bifida could not be excluded until at least 20 weeks' gestation. The couple then asked about the risk to their close family members.

RECURRENCE RISKS

The main individuals at risk within this family are Jeanette and Mark, as they have already conceived one affected child.

Their son, Ethan, is not affected and the risk to his offspring is therefore 1%.

Their siblings, Robert, Sarah and Jason, have a 1% risk of having an affected child.

Sarah's son Kyle's risk of having an affected child is less than 0.5%.

Although there is not an affected living individual in this pedigree, the risk to such an individual of having an affected child would be 3% (i.e. the same as for Jeanette and Mark).

This case illustrates a multifactorial condition present at birth. The risk of occurrence or recurrence can be reduced by taking folic acid in the period immediately before and after conception. In the majority of cases the condition will be detected in the antenatal period by routine screening and the option to terminate an affected foetus is available.

CASE STUDY 2: ADULT ONSET DISORDER

As previously shown, many multifactorial disorders do not present until adult life, and the following case study demonstrates this.

John arranged to see his general practitioner shortly after his brother, Stuart, had a heart attack at the age of 40. Fortunately he survived, but John was aware that several individuals on his father's side of the family had also had heart attacks, and for some this had proved fatal. Both John's parents were well and in their early 70s, and there was no history of heart disease in either his mother's or his wife's families.

CORONARY HEART DISEASE: THE CONDITION

This is a major cause of mortality and morbidity in developed countries, accounting for up to 50% of deaths. It affects both sexes, but is more common in males, and affects all races. It results from atherosclerosis leading to narrowing of the arteries due to deposition of lipid in the arterial wall. The effect on the coronary arteries leads to myocardial ischaemia and, if severe, results in myocardial infarction.

Concordance studies among monozygotic and dizygotic twins has shown an increased incidence among monozygotic twins, suggesting that some genetic factors predispose to this condition, but there are also many environmental factors involved. Evidence for this is in the variation of incidence between different population groups, the incidence in Japan being one sixth of that in Western European countries. Japanese individuals migrating to Western Europe acquire the risk of their new population group within 10–20 years (Mueller & Young, 2001, p. 217).

Genetic factors contributing to coronary heart disease involve multiple genes, including those involved in:

- Cholesterol metabolism.
- Lipid metabolism.
- Blood clotting.

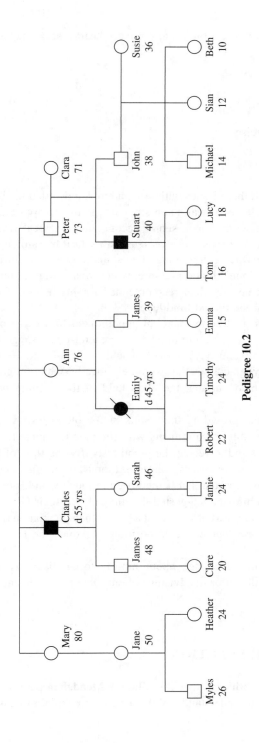

Pedigree 10.2

Environmental factors contributing to coronary heart disease include:

- Smoking.
- Diet high in fats.
- High cholesterol levels.
- Hypertension.
- Insufficient exercise.
- Obesity.
- Stress.

John's GP discussed these issues with him and took a detailed medical and lifestyle history. John, aged 38 years, was a non-smoker with no previous medical or surgical history of note. He worked as a senior accountant in a local firm and described his job as very stressful. His diet was reasonably healthy, although his fat intake tended to be higher when entertaining clients, and he had very little exercise.

The GP checked John's blood pressure, which was within normal limits, and his weight, which was heavier than recommended for his height. The GP also took blood to check cholesterol and lipid levels.

He recommended that John make an appointment to see the practice nurse to discuss diet. He also advised him to take more exercise and suggested that walking to and from work several days a week would be beneficial. He told John about the relaxation and yoga classes that were held locally, which might help to relieve his stress, and pointed out that the class held in the evening had several male participants.

It was agreed that, providing the results of the blood tests were normal, John should have six-monthly appointments with the practice nurse to check his blood pressure and weight and to repeat the blood tests. By the time of his appointment with the practice nurse to discuss diet, his blood test results were available and proved normal. John reported that he had been in touch with his cousins to pass on the advice given to him and suggested that they all see their GPs.

In this situation, John was obviously at a higher than population risk of developing coronary heart disease, but was in a position to reduce the risk by some simple changes to his lifestyle.

With advances in knowledge about multifactorial disorders, the role of the nurse/midwife/health visitor in advising patients about lifestyle changes that reduce risks will increase.

POINTS FOR REFLECTION

- Multifactorial inheritance does not follow a Mendelian pattern. Does this make it more difficult to understand? Will it be easy to explain to patients?

- Knowledge of environmental factors that contribute to disease will become even more important as we recognise genetic factors that predispose individuals to certain disorders.
- How directive should we be when we know there are environmental factors that could be altered to reduce the incidence of a multifactorial disorder in a high-risk family?

REFERENCES

Harper, P.S. (2004) *Practical Genetic Counselling*, 6th edn, Arnold, London.
Connor, M. and Ferguson-Smith, M. (1984) *Essential Medical Genetics*, 5th edn, Blackwell Sciences, Oxford.
Mueller, R.F. and Young, I.D. (eds) (2001) *Emery's Elements of Medical Genetics*, 11th edn, Churchill Livingstone, Edinburgh.

11 Mitochondrial Disorders: Inherited from Mother by Males and Females

JO HAYDON

The modes of inheritance considered in previous chapters have all involved either chromosomes, single genes or a combination of genes, all of which are found in the nucleus of the cell. In contrast to this, mitochondria, containing mitochondrial DNA, are found in the cell cytoplasm. Abnormalities in the mitochondrial DNA can give rise to mitochondrial disorders, which are much less common than chromosome, single gene or multifactorial conditions. A short chapter on mitochondrial inheritance is therefore included for completeness.

Each cell contains hundreds of mitochondria, which are tiny organelles (specialised structures contained with a body cell). They act as power packs for the cell, providing energy for cellular metabolism. They are responsible for processing glucose and oxygen into energy. Many cells use only a small amount of energy and others can use alternative sources to glucose. However, muscle cells use a great deal of energy for movement, and brain cells are not capable of using anything other than glucose for their energy source. When mitochondria are not functioning normally therefore, the most susceptible organs are the central nervous system, skeletal muscles, heart and eyes.

The mitochondria contain DNA which codes for 13 genes, and mutations in these genes may cause serious problems. Cells which contain both normal and abnormal mitochondria may not function as efficiently as normal. Each time such a cell divides, the daughter cells will get a greater or lesser proportion of the mitochondria with an abnormal gene sequence. There can therefore be great variability in the effect of the altered mitochondria, depending on the ratio of normal to abnormal mitochondria within the cell (this is known as heteroplasmy). The variability also depends on the type of tissue or organ affected, as well as the type of change in the sequence of the genetic material. In most mitochondrial disorders, about 75% or more of the mitochondria within a cell must be altered to cause symptoms. This is known as the 'threshold of expression'.

It is possible for an individual to have different proportions of normal and abnormal mitochondria detectable in different samples of blood or other tissues, and the

Genetics in Practice: A clinical approach for healthcare practitioners Edited by Jo Haydon
© 2007 John Wiley & Sons, Ltd

proportions of abnormal mitochondria in one tissue cannot be used to predict the likely proportions in another. The proportion of abnormal mitochondria in the tissues requiring most energy determines the severity of a mitochondrial condition. Prenatal diagnosis is not available for these conditions as the abnormal mitochondria may not be detectable in placental tissue and their presence or absence will not indicate whether the foetus will be affected, nor will it allow any reliable prediction of severity.

COMMON MITOCHONDRIAL CONDITIONS

It should be remembered that mitochondrial conditions are not common, but the following list gives the conditions most often seen:

- Chronic progressive external ophthalmoplegia.
- Diabetes with deafness.
- Hypertrophic cardiomyopathy with myopathy.
- Kearns–Sayre syndrome.
- Leber's hereditary optic neuropathy.
- MELAS syndrome.
- MERFF syndrome.

METHOD OF INHERITANCE

As mitochondria are found in the cytoplasm of the cell, they can only be inherited from the maternal ova, which contain cytoplasm. The cytoplasm in the sperm is contained in the tail, which does not enter the egg at conception. The head of the sperm contains only the nucleus. This means that while both males and females can inherit mitochondrial disorders, they are only inherited from the mother. None of the offspring of an affected male develop any problems.

Different eggs from the same woman will contain different proportions of mitochondrial mutations. Therefore, although all her offspring will inherit her mitochondria, the proportion of mitochondrial mutations will vary, resulting in some offspring becoming affected with the disorder and others remaining clinically unaffected.

When first looking at this pedigree (see Figure 11.2), one might think that it demonstrates a family with a dominant condition as it contains the following features:

- Affected individuals in each generation.
- Males and females roughly equally affected.

But on closer inspection it becomes obvious that:

- There is no male to male or male to female transmission.
- Females may be symptomless carriers.

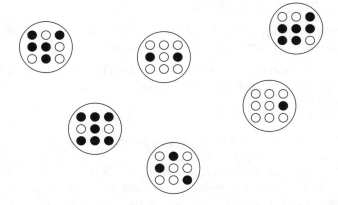

Figure 11.1 Variable Proportions of Mitochondrial Mutations in the Ova

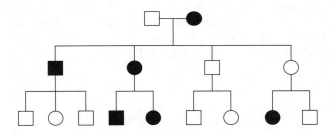

Figure 11.2 A Typical Mitochondrial Pedigree

The proportion of offspring that will become affected is variable (Harper, 2004, p. 48).

Many of the proteins produced in the mitochondria are under the control of gene sequences in the nuclear genome (genes found in the nucleus of the cell). A condition that is associated with defects in the mitochondria may therefore be inherited through a fault in a pair of nuclear genes (usually recessively inherited).

CASE STUDY 1: RISK TO OFFSPRING

Christine was referred for genetic counselling following the diagnosis of MELAS syndrome in her sister, Kathleen. Kathleen, aged 42, was being cared for in a residential home as her family could no longer manage her care needs.

MELAS SYNDROME: THE CONDITION

This is a rare neurodegenerative and fatal disease caused by a mutation in the mitochondrial DNA. The name is an acronym for:

Mitochondrial myopathy, which affects muscles throughout the body
Encephalopathy, causing ataxia, epilepsy and dementia
Lactic **A**cidosis
Stroke-like episodes.

This condition causes a variety of symptoms, many of which are debilitating. Myopathy causes difficulty in walking, moving, eating and speaking. The stroke-like episodes may cause brain damage, leading to epilepsy or partial paralysis. The encephalopathy may cause blindness, deafness and dementia. There is no treatment for the problems associated with the syndrome and the prognosis is poor.

GENETIC COUNSELLING

The genetic counsellor met with Christine, who understood a considerable amount about the syndrome and the poor prognosis for her sister, Kathleen. Christine's main questions were related to the risk to her children. A detailed family tree was drawn up, which showed no other affected individuals.

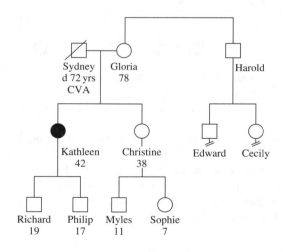

Pedigree 11.1

Kathleen's medical history was also obtained. Kathleen had suffered from epilepsy from the age of 21 years, with the seizures becoming more severe in recent years. She was experiencing hearing problems by the age of 30 and now had a severe hearing loss, making communication very difficult as she had refused to learn signing or lip reading. She had had a stroke several years previously and since that time had become ataxic. Her mental state was thought to be impaired. This was confirmed on MRI scan, when damage in keeping with an infarction was found. Blood tests had revealed high lactate levels and a muscle biopsy had revealed ragged red fibres, a characteristic finding in this condition. A diagnosis of MELAS was suspected and DNA analysis revealed a mutation in the mitochondria.

The GC explained mitochondrial inheritance and Christine was upset to have confirmation that both of Kathleen's sons were at risk but relieved to hear that their offspring could not be affected. At this time they were aged 19 and 14, with no medical problems.

The risk to Christine's children depended on whether or not any evidence of the mutation was found in her mitochondria. Her mother, Gloria, was still alive and well at the age of 78 and had already indicated her willingness to take part in any investigations that might clarify the situation within the family. Blood samples were obtained from both Christine and her mother and the mitochondrial mutation was not found in either sample. Gloria was told that she was unaffected as the likelihood of her developing any symptoms at this late age was negligible. Christine was given a low risk of carrying the gene mutation in other tissue. There was a possibility that Christine could carry the mutation in her germline cells, and if this was the case she might have passed it on to her children. Christine was reassured by the low risk and felt that she would discuss the situation with her children when they were older and give them the option to request testing if they wished.

CASE STUDY 2: MUTATION IN NUCLEAR GENE SUSPECTED AS CAUSE OF MITOCHONDRIAL DISORDER

Susan and Andrew were referred for genetic counselling following the diagnosis of Leigh's disease in their son, James, and daughter, Hannah. James first caused his parents some concern when he was about 15 months old, when he appeared to lose some motor skills and speech. Susan was then eight months pregnant with their second child. Hannah appeared to be normal until the age of 6 months, when she was noted to be losing some skills. The diagnosis of Leigh's disease in both children was made when they were 23 and 7 months old respectively. Blood samples from both children had been obtained in order to examine the mitochondrial DNA and no mutations had been found. At that point their parents were referred for genetic counselling.

LEIGH'S DISEASE: THE CONDITION

Leigh's disease is not a single diagnosis but covers a group of genetic conditions which cause mitochondrial dysfunction. It is a rare neurometabolic disorder characterised by degeneration of the central nervous system. It is a rapidly progressive disorder, with onset usually occurring between the ages of 3 months and 2 years.

The early signs may include poor sucking, loss of head control and loss of previously acquired motor skills. There may be irritability, crying, loss of appetite, vomiting and seizures. As the disease progresses there will be generalised weakness and lack of muscle tone. Lactic acidosis may occur, leading to impaired respiratory and kidney function. Heart problems may also occur. The prognosis is poor, with death usually occurring within a few years. It is an inherited condition and mutations may be identified in either nuclear or mitochondrial genes.

GENETIC COUNSELLING

A detailed family history revealed that Susan's first pregnancy resulted in the birth of a stillborn daughter at 36 weeks' gestation. No obvious cause of death was detected on post mortem. There was no other history of note in either Susan or Andrew's family. Susan and Andrew were first cousins as their fathers were brothers.

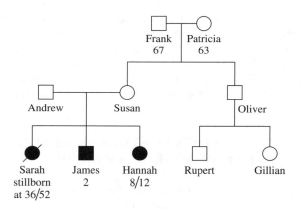

Pedigree 11.2

The geneticist explained that Leigh's disease is not a single diagnosis but covers a group of conditions. He also explained that it could be inherited through mutations in the mitochondria or in the nuclear genes producing mitochondrial enzymes. Susan had no symptoms to suggest that she had the condition and as the tests on the children's mitochondria had been normal, this method of inheritance was thought to be the less likely. Disorders due to faults in the nuclear genes producing mitochondrial enzymes are usually inherited in a recessive fashion and the fact that Susan and Andrew were first cousins added to the likelihood that this was the mode of inheritance in this situation.

On the basis of the information available, the geneticist advised the couple that there was likely to be a 1 in 4 recurrence risk. James was due to have a muscle biopsy in the near future, which might allow identification of the relevant gene fault. The geneticist planned to see the family again in six months' time, when the results of the muscle biopsy would be available.

The results of James's muscle biopsy showed a mutation in the mitochondrial DNA and the same sequence change was found in subsequent blood samples from Hannah and Susan. A further appointment with the geneticist was therefore arranged immediately.

The recurrence risk of 1 in 4 was now revised. Susan and Andrew were told that all future children would inherit Susan's mitochondria and were therefore potentially at risk of being affected. A definite risk figure could not be given but it was thought that it was high as the couple had already had two affected children and it was now suspected that their stillborn daughter might have also been affected.

Susan and Andrew felt that they could not risk this happening again. They already had two seriously affected children whose lifespan was thought to be severely restricted. However, they also wished to pursue any possible options that might lead to the birth of an unaffected child. Prenatal diagnosis would not be reliable and so the possibility of egg donation was discussed. The couple seemed keen to investigate this further and was referred to the assisted conception unit.

Susan's brother, Oliver, was in good health. It was possible that he had the same mitochondrial mutation as Susan but if it was found the effect on his future health, if any, would be unpredictable. Since there was no risk to his offspring, he decided not to be tested. Susan's mother, Patricia, was 63 years old and in good health. Since she had neither siblings nor other daughters there was no practical advantage in offering her a test. Susan was relieved to hear this as she thought her mother would be devastated if the possibility that she had contributed to her grandchildren's illness was even suggested.

Sadly, James died six months later. Hannah was also very ill by this time. The couple was on the waiting list for egg donation and the possibility of this option was a great help to them during this very sad and difficult time in their lives.

POINTS FOR REFLECTION

- When affected males and females are found in several generations, it is important to consider the rules governing mitochondrial inheritance, rather than assuming that the condition is inherited in an autosomal dominant fashion.
- The possibility of mitochondrial inheritance may be avoided by the use of egg donation. However, there are difficulties associated with this procedure.
- Grandparents of an affected child need only be approached for testing if their results will have implications for other family members.

REFERENCE

Harper, P.S. (2004) *Practical Genetic Counselling*, 6th edn, Arnold, London.

12 Cancer Genetics

LUCY BURGESS

In the UK, 1 in 3 of the general population will be affected by cancer during their lifetime (Cancer Research UK, 2003), therefore many people will have an affected family member. Breast, ovarian and colon cancer are particularly common, the incidence of these being:

- Breast: 1 in 9.
- Colon: 1 in 20.
- Ovary: 1 in 48 (Cancer Research UK, 2006).

Most people with cancer will have developed it by chance. However, in some families the pattern of cancers is due to a genetic predisposition. In a small number of these families, genetic testing may be possible.

This chapter aims to help the healthcare professional in their assessment of cancer family histories and their ability to refer patients to the appropriate services as required.

EPIDEMIOLOGY

Most cancer occurs as individuals become older, typically over the age of 65. This is thought to be due to a lifetime of exposure to carcinogens and possibly a reduction in the efficiency of the immune response system. Cancer rarely affects children. There are 1500 cases of childhood cancer diagnosed in the UK each year (Cancer Research UK, 2006). Mortality from cancer accounts for 161, 645 deaths in the UK each year. Survival rates depend on the site, stage, grade and available treatment of the cancer. Over the last 20 years these have improved as detection methods and treatment regimes have improved.

Each year, 10 million cases of cancer are diagnosed worldwide, with different rates occurring in different areas. For example, breast cancer is more common in Northern Europe and America than in Asia and Africa. When assessing family histories, the incidence of cancer within the family may be more significant if

Genetics in Practice: A clinical approach for healthcare practitioners   Edited by Jo Haydon
© 2007 John Wiley & Sons, Ltd

individuals are living in areas where the specific type of cancer is less common. Remember, after several generations, immigrants who adopt the lifestyle of their new community will develop cancer at similar rates to the indigenous population. Boyle *et al.* (Kerr *et al.*, 2001) have highlighted the environmental factors that play a large part in the aetiology of the development of colorectal cancer. They describe the risk of colorectal cancer in adult children of Japanese immigrants to the USA as 3 to 4 times higher than for Japanese individuals living in Japan.

AETIOLOGY

Many environmental factors are known to play a part in the development of cancer. Cancer mainly develops due to a mixture of environmental and genetic factors, but these are not yet well understood. For some people, their lifestyle or carcinogenic exposure is the biggest cancer risk factor, while for others it is their genetic makeup. Only 5–10% of cancers are thought to be due to a known genetic susceptibility. There is no known genetic predisposition that is responsible for all types of cancer, and it is unclear how much difference the modification of lifestyle factors might make to the risk of cancer development for a person who carries a genetic suscep-tibility. When assessing a family history, it is important to consider an individual's medical history, exposure to carcinogens (e.g. at work) and lifestyle factors, as well as possible hereditary factors.

RISK FACTORS

GENERAL

These include diet, alcohol, tobacco, hormones, radiation, viruses and infections, chronic medical conditions and occupational factors.

BREAST CANCER

Breast cancer risk increases with age, 80% of breast cancer occurring over the age of 50. Approximately 1% of breast cancer occurs in men. Having a close relative with breast cancer increases the risk, depending on the age of the affected relative. Other risk factors include delayed childbearing/nulliparity, early menarche/late menopause, prolonged use of HRT, benign breast disease, obesity and radiation to breasts.

COLORECTAL CANCER

Colon cancer risk increases with age and males are more likely to be affected. Again, having a close relative with the disease increases the risk, depending on the age of the relative. Other risk factors include colorectal polyps, chronic disease of the bowel (e.g. Crohn's disease), obesity, alcohol, tobacco and radiation to the pelvic area.

OVARIAN CANCER

Risk factors associated with ovarian cancer include delayed childbearing, infertility, nulliparity/low parity and family history.

INDIVIDUALS AT INCREASED RISK

All cancers are genetic in origin, in that damage to genes is responsible for the development of the cancer. However, only about 5% of patients have cancers that are linked to an inherited gene mutation. About 25% of cancers occur in family clusters and may be due to:

- Other genes that have not yet been discovered.
- Several interacting genes (polygenic).
- Multifactoral mechanisms.
- Environmental/lifestyle factors.
- Chance.

About 75% of cancers probably occur due to chance and/or lifestyle/environmental factors and are therefore sporadic.

Box 12.1 Recognising Significant Family Histories

- Two, three, 3 or more close relatives with the same cancers (e.g. breast, colorectal) in families.
- Early age of onset of cancers.
- Individuals with two or more primary cancers, such as two colorectal primaries, or a bilateral breast cancer.
- Family members with other cancers that could be linked to an inherited colon cancer syndrome, such as endometrial cancer (see HNPCC section) or breast/ovarian cancers.
- Family members with significant lifestyle components (e.g. an affected member exposed to a carcinogen as part of their occupation).

Cole & Sleightholme (2002)

DEVELOPMENT OF CANCER: THE BIOLOGICAL PROCESS

Cancer is a disease in which a normal cell is changed into an invasive malignant cancer cell, and results from ongoing interactions between genes and the environment. Cancer arises from genetic alterations in the DNA, which lead to abnormal cell proliferation. The alteration may arise in the somatic cells of the body or be inherited in the egg or the sperm.

There are several groups of genes which, when altered, have particular involvement in the development of malignant cells:

- Oncogenes, which, when altered, gain function.
- Tumour suppressor genes, which normally act to control cell differentiation and regulate proliferation of cells.
- Gatekeeper genes, which control cell growth and apoptosis (cell death).
- Caretaker genes, which are responsible for helping to control the cell cycle and cell differentiation.

Inherited mutations normally affect tumour suppressor genes, such as BRCA1 and BRCA2 in breast cancer, or the mismatch repair genes in hereditary non-polyposis colon cancer (HNPCC). However, it is important to remember that most individuals who develop cancer do not carry an inherited genetic susceptibility.

AUTOSOMAL DOMINANT INHERITANCE AND TWO-HIT THEORY

Germline mutations which lead to high-risk breast/ovarian cancer (HBOC) families and hereditary non-polyposis colon cancer (HNPCC) are usually inherited in an autosomal dominant manner (see Chapter 7). This means that it only takes one altered copy of the gene for an individual to be susceptible.

However, the mechanism for the development of cancer is slightly different from usual autosomal dominant patterns in that usually the remaining normal copy of a gene pair will be working to provide protection against cancer development. It is only after a second 'hit', caused by an environmental event, that cancer can develop (Knudson, 1996).

Not all individuals who carry an altered gene will develop cancer, due to the genetic phenomenon known as reduced penetrance (see Chapter 7). An individual can be a gene carrier without developing the disease as other mechanisms are at work within the body, such as modifying genes and the influence of the environment. Although the disorder will appear to have skipped a generation, the altered gene has not. In some cancer syndromes, e.g. breast/ovarian cancer, when a BRCA1 mutation is identified, penetrance is 85%, therefore approximately 15% of females with the mutation will not develop cancer.

ASSESSMENT OF FAMILIES WITH A CANCER HISTORY

Many individuals will report having a family history of cancer because cancer is so common. If they meet the referral guidelines (see Table 12.1), they should be offered referral to the local genetics unit or family history service for assessment.

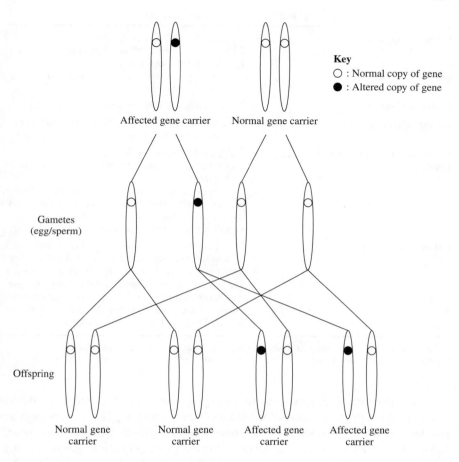

Figure 12.1 Autosomal Dominant Inheritance

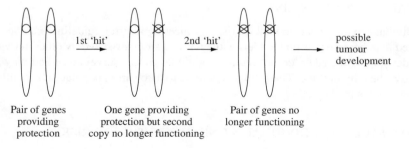

Figure 12.2 Knudson's Two-Hit Theory

Table 12.1 Guidelines for Referral

Breast Cancer	– 1 close relative,* age under 40
	– 1 close relative with bilateral disease
	– 1 male relative, any age
	– 2 close relatives, average** age under 60
	– 3 close relatives, any age
Ovarian Cancer	– 2 close relatives with ovarian cancer, any age
Breast AND Ovarian Cancer	– Minimum of 1 of each cancer; ovarian cancer any age, breast cancer age under 60
Colorectal Cancer (or Colorectal Polyps)	– 1 close relative, age under 45
	– 2 close relatives, average age under 70 (includes both parents)
	– 3 or more close relatives with colorectal cancer or with other gastrointestinal, renal, urinary tract, uterine or ovarian cancer at any age
	– Familial adenomatous polyposis (FAP)
Other cancers	– Multiple primary cancers in one individual
	– 3 or more relatives with cancers at the same site
	– 3 or more relatives with any cancer at an earlier age than expected in the general near-population
	– 3 or more relatives with cancers of breast/ovary/ prostate/pancreas/melanoma/thyroid, or other non-melanoma skin cancers or carcinoma

* Close relatives are: mother/father, sister/brother, son/daughter, aunt/uncle, grandmother/grandfather
** e.g. one relative of 62 and one relative of 56 = an average age of 58

A detailed family history and, following consent from affected individuals, histological confirmation should be obtained where possible. This is important as affected individuals reported to have 'stomach cancer' may be found to have colon, endometrial, ovarian cancers, etc. Once all the relevant information is available, the risk assessment will be made and the appropriate management recommended. The family may be found to be at near-population, moderate or high risk.

NEAR-POPULATION RISK

Individuals with a near-population risk not meeting referral guidelines can be reassured that, based on current evidence, they have a similar risk to any other individual of developing a cancer, do not require additional cancer surveillance and may well enjoy a healthy lifetime. They should continue to take part in population surveillance programmes as they arise.

CASE STUDY 1: INDIVIDUAL AT NEAR POPULATION RISK

Michelle visited her practice nurse for her regular cervical smear. While there, she asked if she had an increased risk of cancer as her mother had been treated for a skin cancer at the age of 59 and her maternal grandmother died from a breast cancer in her 80s. No other family members had had cancer as far as she was aware.

Her practice nurse checked her history against the referral guidelines. She was able to reassure Michelle that the cancers were most likely due to chance as they had occurred in older individuals. Michelle added that her mother had always loved to sunbathe and that she had not used skin protection until recently.

The practice nurse suggested to Michelle that she should be breast aware and report any untoward signs and symptoms to her GP, should follow healthy lifestyle advice, use skin protection and continue to take part in population cancer surveillance programmes as appropriate.

The practice nurse also suggested that Michelle check that her aunt, Hilda, was on the National Breast Screening programme.

Michelle was satisfied with the advice given and decided to learn a bit more about the signs and symptoms of cancer by looking on the web site www.cancerhelp. org.uk, which the practice nurse had recommended.

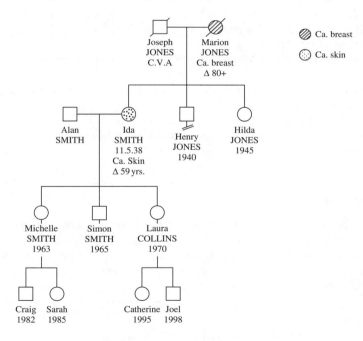

Pedigree 12.1 Near-population Risk

MODERATE RISK

Those individuals in moderate risk categories can be seen by the relevant healthcare professional, either a member of the genetic staff or a nurse specialist in the local hospital, for an explanation of their risk and recommendations for surveillance. The healthcare professional should:

- Explore the patient's past medical history, checking for symptoms, e.g. rectal bleeding, for which urgent investigations may be required.
- Obtain information regarding occupation, lifestyle, anxieties and worries.
- Extend the pedigree where necessary to ensure that all close relatives are included, affected and unaffected, living and dead. This ensures that all individuals requiring surveillance either now or at a later date are recognised.
- Clarify information about cancers, e.g. age at diagnosis, whether the breast cancer was bilateral or a recurrence. Include other available details, e.g. grade, hormonal status and treatment of breast cancer.
- Obtain as much information about unconfirmed types of cancer as possible, including age of cancer occurrence.
- Record ethnicity.
- Discuss screening type, frequency and limitations of surveillance.
- Consider storing or asking for consent from relatives to store a DNA sample (see Box 12.2), or ask for consent for tumour block studies if dealing with an abdominal cancer family.
- Discuss relevant lifestyle and health recommendations based on relevant research.
- Reassure the individual that it is still more likely that they will not develop a cancer than that they will.
- Discuss any other concerns related to the family history.
- Ask to be informed if other family information comes to light so that the risk can be reassessed.

Box 12.2 DNA Banking

- May be suggested when a genetic test is not yet available but research in the appropriate area is underway.
- Consent is obtained to obtain a blood sample from an affected patient or a relative with cancer in a moderate or high-risk family.
- DNA is extracted and stored.

CASE STUDY 2: MODERATE RISK FAMILY

Julie approached her GP for advice when her maternal aunt was found to have breast cancer, as her own mother had had breast cancer at the age of 50. The GP referred her to the clinical genetics unit for advice and Julie's risk of breast cancer was assessed to be approximately 18% over her lifetime. Therefore it was still much more likely that she would not develop a breast cancer than that she would. However, it was suggested that she be breast aware and seek advice regarding the latest breast surveillance recommendations when she approached the age of 40 (NICE, 2006). The same advice applied to her four sisters and her aunt's two daughters. She was also advised to continue with regular cervical smears as her sister had had cervical cancer. However, this was not thought to be connected to the family history of breast cancer.

It was important that Julie was aware of the limitations of breast surveillance, including the facts that breast cancers can occur between breast screens and that benign changes may be detected which require further investigations, such as a biopsy, and that this may cause undue worry (Moss, 2004). Routine breast surveillance is not recommended for women under the age of 35 as their breasts are more dense than those of older women and thus more difficult to visualise on mammography. Also, theoretically, as mammograms use X-rays there is a risk of causing damage to the DNA of the breast cells and possibly causing cancerous changes (Lucassen *et al.*, 2001). Mammography has been shown to reduce mortality in the 50–64 age group (Blanks *et al.*, 2000), but screening of younger women is not as yet supported by evidence and is the subject of ongoing research.

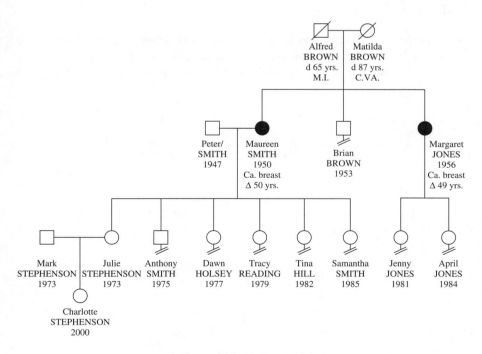

Pedigree 12.2 Moderate Risk

CASE STUDY 3: ALTERED RISK ON FURTHER INVESTIGATION

Kevin's sister, Maureen, was thought to have had bowel cancer at the age of 39 and Kevin's GP referred him for regular colonoscopies. When he was seen in the genetics centre, the cancer intelligence records for Maureen showed that she had in fact had an ovarian cancer. Therefore Kevin was at population risk of bowel cancer and would not require bowel surveillance.

HIGH RISK

Any family at high risk of developing breast, ovarian, colorectal or other associated cancers will usually be seen by the cancer clinical geneticist and/or genetic counsellor. Genetic testing may be possible, using DNA from an affected family member. This will involve obtaining a blood sample or using stored DNA. In either case, the family member whose DNA is to be tested should be seen to discuss the implications of the test, both for themselves and for other family members. This may be particularly important if another family member, e.g. a niece or nephew, has instigated the referral. It is important to ensure that the affected individual does not feel under pressure to provide a blood sample for analysis. Genetic counselling may help to clarify the individual's feelings and anxieties and identify coping strategies to deal with the test results.

If a gene alteration is found:

- The affected individual may be at increased risk of developing other cancers and should be aware of any available surveillance and/or risk-reducing surgery.
- The offspring of that individual will be at 50% risk of having inherited the gene alteration.

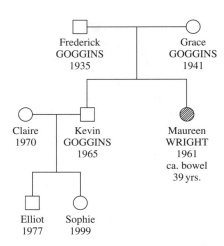

Pedigree 12.3 Original Pedigree

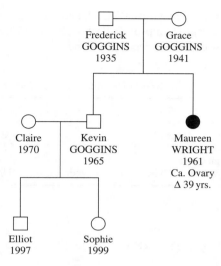

Pedigree 12.4 Pedigree after Histological Confirmation

- Predictive testing will be available to other at-risk family members (see Chapter 5) and those found to carry the gene alteration should be offered the appropriate surveillance.
- If an at-risk individual decides not to have the predictive test, surveillance should continue.
- If the individual is tested and does not carry the gene alteration, their risk returns to that of the general population and additional screening will not be required.

If a gene alteration is not found:

- This does not mean that the family history is not caused by a gene alteration, only that the alteration is not currently identifiable. As genetic knowledge increases and laboratory techniques become more sophisticated, identification may become possible at a future date.
- The risk to offspring and other family members is not altered.
- Predictive testing will not be available to family members, who will be encouraged to continue with appropriate surveillance.

BREAST/OVARIAN CANCER FAMILIES

A strong family history of cancer may be caused by a specific gene mutation in a family and there are thought to be many different gene mutations that will increase breast/ovarian cancer risk. At present, two specific gene alterations have been identified. These are known as BRCA1 and BRCA2 and account for about 5–10% of all breast cancer (Thompson & Easton, 2004). There are on-going studies to identify other breast cancer susceptibility genes.

Table 12.2 Genes Involved in Hereditary Breast Cancer Syndromes

Condition	Gene
Hereditary breast cancer	BRCA1 BRCA2
Li Fraumeni syndrome	p53
Ataxia telangiectasia	ATM
Cowden's syndrome (PTEN mutation syndromes)	PTEN

GENES ASSOCIATED WITH BREAST CANCER

BRCA1

This gene is found on chromosome 17q21 and its altered form is thought to account for about 15–45% of hereditary breast cancers. This gene normally acts as a tumour suppressor gene. Women who have inherited a BRCA1 mutation have:

- Up to 85% risk of developing breast cancer over their lifetime.
- 40–60% risk of a second primary breast cancer.
- Up to 60% risk of developing an ovarian cancer.
- An increased risk of pancreatic, fallopian tube and cervical cancer.

BRCA1 mutations are found most frequently in patients with medullary breast cancer and those who have oestrogen receptor-negative cancers. Breast cancer in BRCA1 carriers is most likely to be a grade 3, oestrogen receptor-negative cancer.

Males carrying the BRCA1 mutation have a slightly increased risk of prostate cancer (Thompson & Easton, 2002).

BRCA2

BRCA2 is found on chromosome 13q12. Women who have inherited a BRCA2 mutation have:

- Up to 85% risk of developing breast cancer over their lifetime.
- 40–60% risk of a second primary breast cancer.
- 10–20% risk of developing ovarian cancer.
- An increased risk of pancreatic, bile duct, gall bladder and stomach cancers and malignant melanoma.

Men who carry a BRCA2 mutation have:

- Up to 6% risk of developing breast cancer, and should be aware of breast changes, which they should report to their doctor.
- An increased risk of about 20% of developing prostate cancer.

Males with a family history of breast cancer may be worried about the risk to themselves and their daughters.

Box 12.3 Ethnic Origin Related to BRCA1 and BRCA2

- Ashkenazi Jews have a higher risk of inheriting breast cancers and these families do not need to meet the minimum referral guidelines for referral.
- Genetic testing may be available for unaffected individuals even if there are no living family members. Amongst Ashkenazi Jews there are three specific mutations, two in BRCA1 and one in BRCA2.

OPTIONS AVAILABLE TO WOMEN IN HIGH-RISK FAMILIES

There are a number of options available to women in high-risk families. The choices that such women make will depend on their previous experience of cancer. A woman who has seen her relatives die from cancer at a very young age may be more likely to seek prophylactic surgery than someone whose relatives have been treated successfully.

Surveillance

A comprehensive screening programme is recommended. Women should be aware of changes in their breasts and have access to their local breast service. Clinical examinations may be offered from around the age of 25, although this has not been proven to reduce mortality. However, Burke et al. (1997) report that approximately 10% of breast cancers may be detected by this method. Mammography is offered from around the age of 35 (Eccles et al., 2000), but this does not detect all cancers and benign conditions may require ongoing investigations. MRI may be offered to high-risk and BRCA-positive women from the age of 30 (NICE, 2006). Although this has a high sensitivity, it has a low specificity and the frequent detection of benign lesions may cause unnecessary anxiety. The advantage is that the procedure, although expensive, does not involve the use of radiation, which may be of particular importance to younger women, where the potential risk of increased radiation exposure is greatest.

BRCA1 and BRCA2 carriers who have had breast cancer are at increased risk of a second primary breast cancer and the lifetime risk may be as great as 60% (Easton et al., 1995). It is important that affected women who have had breast conserving surgery are not discharged from follow-up and continue to have annual mammography. Some affected women may wish to consider contralateral mastectomy.

Prophylactic Mastectomy

Bilateral prophylactic mastectomy can reduce breast cancer risk by 90% (Hartmann *et al.*, 1999) in women with BRCA1 and BRCA2 mutations, depending on the type of surgery performed. Women who request prophylactic mastectomy should have genetic counselling, confirmation of family history, psychological assessment and pre-operative evaluation by breast care nurses and surgeons (Meijers-Heijboer *et al.*, 2000) as the psychological consequences of this procedure can be variable. Management should be in units with a structured care pathway (NICE, 2006). The use of chemoprevention agents such as tamoxifen is the subject of ongoing research and these are not yet licensed for use in this risk group in the UK (Cusick *et al.*, 2003).

Ovarian Surveillance, Chemoprevention and Surgical Options

Ovarian cancer with a genetic predisposition may not necessarily occur at a younger age, unlike other cancers with a genetic predisposition. The oral contraceptive pill is protective against the development of ovarian cancer (Narod *et al.*, 1998). Women in high risk groups are offered annual transvaginal ultrasound (TVS) with colour Doppler imaging and CA-125 II analysis, starting at around the age of 35. CA-125 is a tumour marker; levels can rise when ovarian cancer is present. However, levels can also rise when there are inflammatory changes in the abdomen and therefore CA-125 II analysis has low specificity. The usefulness of TVS in screening high-risk women is unproven (Rosenthal & Jacobs, 1998) and is the subject of an ongoing study (UKFOCSS).

Prophylactic salpingo-oophrectomy may be requested by women because of the limitations of surveillance. It reduces the risk of ovarian cancer by 95%. It is important that the fallopian tubes are removed, especially in BRCA1 carriers (Sobal *et al.*, 2000). Additionally, bilateral salpingo-oophrectomy reduces the risk of breast cancer by between a third and a half (Rebbeck *et al.*, 1999) if performed before the menopause. Women should consider issues of fertility, cancer risk, hormone replacement therapy (which is not contraindicated before the natural age of the menopause), the menopause and the type of surgery in detail when considering prophylactic surgery.

CASE STUDY 4: HIGH-RISK FAMILY HISTORY

Mandy's mother, Judy, had died from an ovarian cancer at the age of 48. Her mother's oncologist suggested that the family should ask advice about the family history. Mandy had reached the age of 40 and worried that she might develop ovarian cancer too. She was referred to the clinical genetics unit and, on completing a family history form, realised that there was also a family history of breast cancer. Her aunt, Glynis, had had breast cancer at the age of 39, and her grandmother at the age of 40. The family was assessed as high risk and Mandy and her siblings were offered a genetic clinic appointment. The genetic counsellor discussed the family tree and suggested that genetic testing for BRCA1 or BRCA2 alterations could be offered to Glynis. In the meantime she arranged for Mandy, her sister, Charlotte, and her cousin, Anna (Glynis's daughter), to commence annual breast and ovarian screening.

The GC spoke to Glynis, who was keen to undergo genetic testing because of her worries about her children. The GC discussed the implications of testing for Glynis, including her increased risk of a second primary breast cancer and ovarian cancer if a mutation was found. Blood was taken and sent to the genetic molecular laboratories and a mutation in Glynis's BRCA1 gene was identified. This meant that there was a 50% risk that Anna and Adam had inherited the altered gene. They were aware that they could request a genetic test to clarify their situation but felt that they needed time to consider this option.

Glynis's result suggested that it was likely that Judy had had the same gene alteration, and therefore Mandy and her siblings may have inherited it. After a further counselling session, Mandy decided to have a genetic test, which showed that she did not carry the altered BRCA1 gene. She now had a population risk of developing breast cancer and her extra screening was no longer necessary. Her brother, Adam,

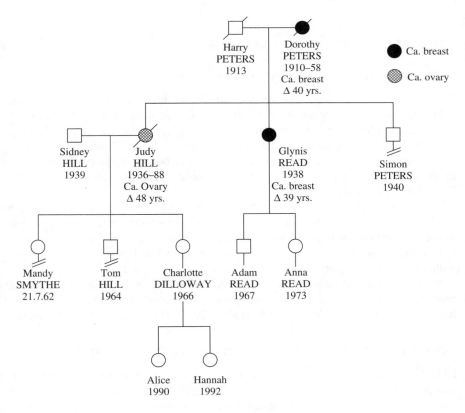

Pedigree 12.5

unfortunately tested positive for the gene alteration. This meant that his risk for prostate cancer was slightly increased and prostate surveillance, in the form of PSA testing and digital rectal examination, was suggested, starting in his 40s. Mandy's sister, Charlotte, did not want to have the genetic test as she felt that she would worry too much if she was found to carry the gene alteration. She was pleased to hear that despite this she would be offered annual breast and ovarian surveillance.

Glynis's brother, Simon, was also potentially at risk of having inherited the gene alteration. He did not wish to proceed with testing and also declined prostate surveillance.

Glynis commenced annual mammograms and had her ovaries removed. She felt that identifying the altered gene in the family has been a positive experience as it gave her children, nieces and nephew more opportunity to be proactive about their health. She felt hopeful that the extra surveillance would help identify any cancers at an earlier and more curable stage. She also agreed to take part in a research trial looking at lifestyle risk factors and their effect on the development of disease in BRCA1 and BRCA2 carriers.

COLORECTAL CANCER FAMILIES

FAMILIAL ADENOMATOUS POLYPOSIS (FAP)

This is an autosomal dominant genetic condition which causes about 1% of all colorectal cancers. Individuals who carry the altered gene develop hundreds of adenomatous polyps, and if they remain untreated, colorectal cancer will develop (Burlow, 1987). The condition is described in more detail in Chapter 7.

Attenuated FAP is a variation of FAP with fewer polyps developing and a later onset of cancer. Not all individuals with the gene alteration will develop cancer (incomplete penetrance).

An alteration in the APC gene which has been identified in about 6% of the Ashkenazi Jewish population doubles their risk of colorectal cancer. It is important to ascertain ethnic background to determine if genetic testing for this alteration is appropriate, as in this population testing this can be undertaken in a family member without the need to analyse the DNA of an affected individual.

Individuals without features of classical FAP but with several adenomas may have a recessively inherited condition, increasing the risk of bowel cancer (MutYH). For the individual to be susceptible, they need an altered copy of the gene from both parents.

HEREDITARY NON-POLYPOSIS COLORECTAL CANCER (HNPCC)

HNPCC is a condition in which polyps can occur in the bowel (despite the term non-polyposis). There may be a fairly rapid progression to colorectal cancer. Other cancers may also occur, including renal tract transitional cell carcinoma, ovarian cancer, small bowel adenoma and endometrial cancer.

Table 12.3 Approximate Rates of Incidence of Cancer in HNPCC

Cancer	Approximate incidence in HNPCC%
Colorectal cancer:	
Males aged 50 and 70	45 and 70
Females aged 50 and 70	20 and 35
Endometrial age 50 and 70	10 and 40
Small bowel adenocarcinoma	1–2
Stomach	1–12
Ovarian	10
Bladder	Less than 10
Renal	Less than 10

Because of the variety of cancers that may occur, it is useful to have some guidelines for identifying HNPCC families. Syngal *et al.* (2000) suggest that if the modified Amsterdam criteria (Table 12.4) are used then HNPCC represents 3–5% of colorectal cancers.

Table 12.4 Modified Amsterdam II Criteria

Three or more cases of colorectal or associated cancer
A minimum of two generations affected
One first degree relative of the other two affected
One case diagnosed before the age of 50
FAP excluded

Mutations in genes causing these cancers have been identified in the mismatch repair genes MLH1, MSH2, MSH6, PMS1 and PMS2. Genetic testing is currently routinely available for MLH1, MSH2 and NSH6. Testing for other genes involved may be available on a research basis.

Guidelines for screening in HNPCC families will depend on the types of cancer found within a particular family. Burt (2000) suggests that recommendations for surveillance other than colonoscopy vary widely and will depend on individual family histories.

OPTIONS AVAILABLE TO INDIVIDUALS IN HIGH-RISK FAMILIES

Colon Screening

Colorectal cancer can be detected by colonoscopy, which has been proven to be of benefit (Dove-Edwin *et al.*, 2005) in reducing mortality from the disease. Guidelines for bowel screening recommend the use of colonosocopy because of the incidence of right-sided tumours in high-risk families (Levin *et al.*, 1999). The recommended frequency of screening is 1–3 yearly, commencing at 25–30, depending on family history, actual risk, available resources and local guidelines (Burt, 2000). Occasionally, prophylactic colectomy may be considered by some asymptomatic gene mutation carriers (Vasen *et al.*, 1996). The change from adenoma to carcinoma may take only 1–2 years. However, Wijnen *et al.* (1998) suggest that prognosis is better in individuals with HNPCC than for those with sporadic colorectal cancers.

Colonoscopy requires full bowel preparation and sedation is usually given. The endoscopist is able to see the whole of the mucosal lining of the colon and to remove any small polyps seen. However, patients may find the bowel preparation unpleasant, leading to non-compliance, which will reduce the ability to fully examine the bowel. The procedure does not allow visualisation of the caecum. Patients may be anxious and fearful regarding the procedure, leading to non-attendance. They may also find the procedure embarrassing or distasteful. Occasionally, if there is a real fear of the procedure, virtual colonoscopy in the form of CT scanning may be a possibility. Complications include the possibility of over sedation or under sedation, leading to pain and discomfort. In addition, there is a 1 in 6000 risk of bowel perforation.

Gynaecological Screening

Women who are HNPCC gene carriers are at a 60% lifetime risk of developing endometrial cancer and may therefore have a greater risk of developing endometrial cancer than colon cancer. Annual transvaginal ultrasound and hysteroscopy/endometrial biopsy may be recommended, although Cole & Sleigtholme (2002) argue that there is little evidence to support this programme because the survival rate from endometrial cancer is high and routine surveillance may not alter the detection rate. Transvaginal ultrasound (and CA-125 measurements) may be of benefit in assessment of the ovaries, as ovarian cancer incidence is also increased in HNPCC carriers. Evidence to support this surveillance procedure is also lacking. Some female gene carriers may opt for hysterectomy and bilateral oophrectomy around the age of the menopause as this will substantially reduce their risk of developing endometrial or ovarian cancer.

Other Surveillance

Other surveillance may be recommended, such as urological or gastric surveillance, depending on the family history.

Chemoprevention

Evidence is emerging that aspirin, resistant starch, NSAIDs and Cox 2 inhibitors have an effect on slowing down the growth of colorectal cancer in FAP and HNPCC patients (Huls *et al.*, 2003).

Cancer Tissue Studies

Tumour tissue from patients who developed colorectal cancer under the age of 35 or who had a moderate or strong family history of colorectal cancer may be examined to look for micro-satellite instability. This unstable factor can contribute to the development of cancer and the type and extent of the changes may help in the future with understanding diagnosis and treatment of the disease.

If micro-satellite instability is identified, there is a greatly increased likelihood that MSH1 or MLH2 gene alterations will be found in the DNA from a blood sample (Farrington *et al.*, 1998).

Immunohistochemistry (IHC) analysis can also be undertaken on cancer tissue. If there is an absence of staining with antibodies of the MLH1, MSH2 or MSH6 proteins, this helps target which one of the HNPCC genes to analyse first in an individual.

Table 12.5 Genes Involved in Hereditary Bowel Cancer Syndromes

Condition	Gene
Peutz-Jegher syndrome	STK11
Turcot's syndrome	MMR genes
Cowden's syndrome (PTEN mutation syndromes)	PTEN
Juvenile polyposis	SMAD4

CASE STUDY 5: USE OF CANCER TISSUE STUDIES

Sally's brother Richard had colon cancer at the age of 54. Their father had colon cancer at the age of 72 and his sister had endometrial cancer at the age of 66. Sadly all three affected relatives with cancer had died. Sally consented to tumour tissue studies on her brother's cancer tissue, stored in the histopathology department of the hospital where Richard was treated. The IHC results indicated an absence of staining for MSH2 proteins and MSI studies indicated micro-satellite instability. These results meant that this was likely to be an HNPCC family and it was estimated that Sally's risk of bowel and endometrial cancer was increased. Sally was therefore advised to have 3-yearly bowel surveillance and annual gynaecological surveillance.

This chapter has concentrated on the more common inherited cancers. The genetic study of cancer will increase our understanding of the aetiology, management and treatment of cancer. In the future, genetic markers may lead to better identification of those at high risk of the disease, who can then be offered regular surveillance, leading to earlier diagnosis and treatment.

POINTS FOR REFLECTION

- 1 in 3 people in the general population will develop cancer and therefore most cases will be sporadic.
- The known cancer susceptibility genes account for less than 50% of inherited cancers.

- Predictive genetic testing is usually only possible after the identification of a specific gene mutation in an affected family member and is difficult to undertake unless there is a living affected family member or DNA has been banked from an affected person. However, more recently in very high risk families, indirect genetic testing (testing three or more closely related unaffected individuals) may be considered.
- How might you sensitively raise the issue of obtaining a DNA sample, for future benefit to the family, with a terminally ill patient?

REFERENCES

Blanks, R.G. *et al.* (2000) Effect of NHS screening programme on mortality from breast cancer in England and Wales 1990–8: Comparison of observed with predicted mortality. *BMJ*, **321**, 665–9.

Burke, W. *et al.* (1997) Recommendations for follow-up care of individuals with inherited predisposition to cancer. *JAMA*, **237**(12), 997–1003.

Burlow, S. (1987) Familial adenomatous polyposis. *Danish Medical Journal*, **34**, 1–15.

Burt, R.W. (2000) Colon cancer screening . *Gastroenterology*, **119**, 837–53.

Cancer Research UK (2003) Cancer stats. Available at: info.cancerresearchuk.org/cancer stats.

Cancer Research UK (2006) Available at: http://info.cancerresearchuk.org/cancerstats/.

Cole, T.R.P. and Sleigtholme, H.V. (2002) ABC of colorectal cancer: the role of clinical genetics in management. *British Medical Journal*, **321**, 1779–80.

Cusick, J. *et al.* (2003) Overview of the main outcomes in breast-cancer prevention trials. *Lancet*, **361**, 296–300.

Dove-Edwin, I. *et al.* (2005) Prevention of colorectal cancer by colonoscopic surveillance in individuals with a family history of colorectal cancer: 16 year, prospective follow-up study. *BMJ*, **331**(7524), 1047.

Easton, D., Ford, D. and Bishop, T.D. (1995) Breast Cancer Linkeage Consortium: Breast and ovarian cancer incidence in BRCA1 carriers. *American Journal of Human Genetics*, **56**, 265–71.

Eccles, D., Evans, D.G. and Makay, J. (2000) Guidelines for a genetic risk based approach advising women with a family history of breast cancer. *Journal of Medical Genetics*, **37**(3), 203–9.

Eeles, R.A. (2004) *Genetic Predisposition to Cancer*, 2nd edn, Arnold, New York.

Farrington, S.M. *et al.* (1998) Systematic analysis of mis-match repair genes in colon cancer patients and controls. *American Journal of Human Genetics*, **63**, 749–59.

Hartmann, L.C. *et al.* (1999) Efficacy of bilateral prophylactic mastectomy in women with a family history of breast cancer. *The New England Journal of Medicine*, **340**(2), 77–84.

Huls, G., Koornstra, J.J. and Kleibeuker, J.H. (2003) Non-steroidal anti-inflammatory drugs and molecular carcinogenesis of colorectal carcinomas. *Lancet*, **362**, 230–2.

Kerr, D.J., Young, A.M. and Hobbs, F.D.R. (eds) (2001) ABC of Colorectal Cancer, *British Medical Journal*, London.

Knudson, A.G. (1996) Hereditary cancer: Two hits revisited. *Journal of Cancer Research and Clinical Oncology*, **122**, 135–40.

Levin, T.R. *et al.* (1999) Predicting advanced proximal colonic neoplasia with screening sigmoidoscopy. *JAMA*, **281**, 1611–17.

Lucassen, A. *et al.* (2001) Advice about mammography for a young women with a family history of cancer. *British Medical Journal*, **322**, 1040–2.

Meijers-Heijboer, E.J. *et al.* (2000) Presymptomatic DNA testing and prophylactic surgery in families with a BRCA1 and BRCA2 mutation. *Lancet*, **355**(9220), 2015–20.

Moss, S. (2004) Screening for breast cancer in high risk populations. In: *Genetic Predisposition to Cancer* (Eeles, R.A.), 2nd edn, Arnold, New York.

Narod, S.A. *et al.* (1998) Oral contraceptives and the risk of hereditary ovarian cancer. *NEJM*, **339**(7), 424–8.

NICE (2006) *Familial Breast Cancer: Nice Guideline CG014*, London.

Rebbeck, T.R. *et al.* (1999) Breast cancer risk after bilateral prophylactic oophrectomy in BRCA1 mutation carriers. *Journal of the National Cancer Institute*, **91**, 1475–9.

Rosenthal, A. and Jacobs, I. (1998) Ovarian cancer screening: Seminars. *Oncology*, **25**(3), 315–25.

Sobal, H. *et al.* (2000) Fallopian tube cancer as a feature of BRCA1: Associated syndromes. *Gynecological Oncology*, **78**, 263–6.

Syngal, S. *et al.* (2000) Sensitivity and specificity of clinical criteria for hereditary non-polyposis colorectal cancer associated mutations in MSH2 and MLH1. *Journal of Medical Genetics*, **37**, 641–5.

Thompson, D. and Easton, D. (2002) Cancer incidence in BRCA1 mutation carriers. *Journal of the National Cancer Institute*, **94**(18), 1358–65.

Thompson, D. and Easton, D. (2004) The BRCA1 and BRCA2. In: *Genetic Predisposition to Cancer* (Eeles, R.A.), 2nd edn, Arnold, New York.

UKFOCSS (UK Familial Ovarian Cancer Screening Study) (year unknown) Unpublished trial.

Vasen, H.F., Watson, P., Mecklin, J.P. *et al.* (1996) New clinical criteria for hereditary nonpolyposis colorectal cancer (HNPCC, Lynch syndrome) proposed by the International Collaborative Group on HNPCC. Gastroenterology, 110, 1020–7.

Wijnen, J.T. *et al.* (1998) Clinical findings with implications for genetic testing in families with clustering of colorectal cancer. *New England Journal of Medicine*, **339**, 511–18.

13 Ethnicity

JO HAYDON

The term 'ethnicity' may be used to refer to 'socially constructed differences, grounded in culture, ancestry and language rather than in supposed physical or geological differences' (Culley & Dyson, 2001, p. 40). Culture is 'a shared set of norms, values, assumptions and perceptions (both explicit and implicit) and social conventions which enable members of a group ... to function cohesively' (Schott & Henley, 1996, p. 3) and may be regarded as the total way of life of an individual. Many of the components of an individual's culture are absorbed during childhood from the family and community within which the individual lives. They are regarded as the norm and will influence decisions made throughout life.

Britain is a multicultural society but it is easy to forget the many similarities that exist between the various cultures that make up this country and to focus on the differences. If we are to respect other cultures we need to be aware of our own cultural values and beliefs and recognise their importance to our sense of self. We should be aware of the beliefs and values of other cultures so that we are able to treat individuals from these cultures with respect. It is essential to refrain from stereotyping individuals or assume that because an individual is of a certain nationality or religion they will share all the values associated with that grouping. We must also recognise that for some people, religious belief and personal practice will not always be the same.

In the next section, some of the factors that can influence the decisions made by families with a genetic condition will be considered.

OVERVIEW OF CULTURAL DIFFERENCES

COMMUNICATION

Communication involves far more than the use of language. The way that we use language also helps to convey meaning. Our use of intonation, emphasis and timing can indicate politeness or anger, aggression or resentment. The volume that we use may be interpreted differently between cultures. We use non-verbal clues such as

Genetics in Practice: A clinical approach for healthcare practitioners Edited by Jo Haydon
© 2007 John Wiley & Sons, Ltd

eye contact, facial expressions, physical proximity, gestures and touch to convey meaning. However, these have different interpretations in different cultures. In European cultures, eye contact is regarded as a sign of trustworthiness, whereas in Asian cultures it may be regarded as aggression and in African-Caribbean cultures, as a sign of insolence. In some cultures it is inappropriate to touch someone of the opposite sex, and close physical proximity may be regarded similarly. Each culture assumes that its own behaviour is correct, so professionals need to have some awareness of the variations they may encounter.

Level of understanding can be difficult to assess when a client speaks some English but is not fluent in the language. It may be necessary to ask questions during the consultation to help clarify this. When individuals being seen do not understand English, the use of an interpreter may be necessary. However, this is not always a straightforward matter. When an interpreter is used for a genetic counselling consultation they must be aware of the sensitivity of the discussion and the need not to convey their own feelings about the issues being discussed. The interpreter may need some preparation beforehand to understand the terminology being used. The client may be reluctant to discuss sensitive subjects with an interpreter, whom they may wrongly regard as not being bound by the same professional rules of confidentiality as the genetic counsellor. Sometimes an interpreter will be known to the family if they are from the same community, and this can increase the concerns of the clients, cause embarrassment and lead to restrictions in the disclosure of information. If a relative is asked to interpret, they may not give all the information to the client if they want to protect them from bad news or do not believe it themselves. Under no circumstances should children be asked to interpret for their parents as this is inappropriate and likely to cause embarrassment or refusal to disclose/discuss information of a highly personal nature.

The ideal situation is to have genetic counsellors who are fluent in the languages of the most common non-English speaking population in an area, and in some regions with high Pakistani populations this practice has been established. However, with the increase in immigration from Eastern European and other parts of the world (e.g. Somalia), there are many more languages for which interpreters are needed.

FAMILY RELATIONSHIPS AND DECISION MAKING

When a genetic condition is diagnosed in an individual, members of their extended family can be faced with difficult decisions. If professionals are going to help in facilitating decision-making, they need to be aware of possible cultural differences in how decisions are reached within a family, as patterns of authority may differ.

In some cultures, men are regarded as the prime decision makers. In other cultures, a couple may defer to older family members to make decisions for them. In yet other cultures with strong matriarchal biases, the older women in the family will be dominant.

CONSANGUINITY

This refers to the practice of marriage between related individuals (second cousins or closer) and is practiced by about 17% of the world population, with more than 20% of all marriages being consanguineous (Bittles, 1998). The majority of such marriages are between first cousins. Consanguineous marriage is favoured throughout the Middle East and in much of South Asia, some parts of Sub-Saharan Africa and South East Asia, and among some Jewish communities and Irish Travellers. In the past it was widely practiced among the British aristocracy. Consanguinity is also common in remote, isolated communities throughout the world.

The incidence of consanguinity is greater among members of certain religions, e.g. Muslims, the Dravidian Hindus of South India. Other religions absolutely prohibit marriages between cousins, e.g. Sikhs and Aryan Hindus. Among Roman Catholics, marriage of first cousins is only allowed with special dispensation. First-cousin marriages may also be restricted by national legislation and are criminal offences in 8 states in the USA and illegal in a further 31 states (Ottenheimer, 1990).

Among those who practice it, consanguineous marriage may be a strong family tradition and confer social benefits. These include the strengthening of family ties by the retention of land and property, and reduction of the need for a large dowry. Consanguineous marriage is also thought to provide greater protection for women as they are already a member of their husband's family and a niece of their parents-in-law. There is a lower incidence of divorce. Following immigration, marriage to a relative can help prevent feelings of cultural isolation.

However, consanguinity is associated with an increased risk of autosomal recessive disease as the number of ancestors from whom genes are inherited is smaller (i.e. there is a smaller ancestral gene pool).

If an individual's parents are unrelated (Figure 13.1), they will have:

- Two parents.
- Four grandparents.
- Eight great-grandparents.
- Sixteen great-great-grandparents.

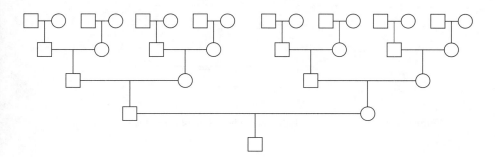

Figure 13.1 Ancestors of an Individual whose Parents are Unrelated

If an individual's parents are first cousins (Figure 13.2), they will have:

- Two parents.
- Four grandparents.
- Six great-grandparents.
- Twelve great-great-grandparents.

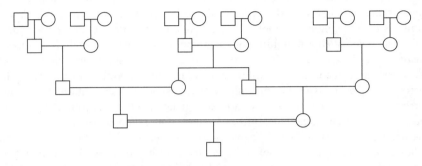

Figure 13.2 Ancestors of an Individual whose Parents are First Cousins

If an individual's parents are double first cousins (Figure 13.3), they will have:

- Two parents.
- Four grandparents.
- Four great-grandparents.
- Eight great-great-grandparents.

This individual will have only half as many great-great-grandparents as an individual whose parents are not related.

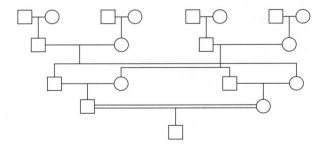

Figure 13.3 Ancestors of an Individual whose Parents are Double First Cousins

We all carry several gene alterations for autosomal recessive disorders but this is only a problem if our partner carries an alteration in the same gene and both partners pass on the gene alteration to their offspring (see Chapter 8). The more common ancestors that we have, the greater the risk of this happening. However, it is important not to overemphasise this risk. The risk to any first-cousin couple, where there is no known autosomal recessive condition in the family, is 2–3% above the population risk.

When recording a family history, it is always important to ask about consanguinity, regardless of an individual's nationality, as this may be important in assessing the risk to offspring. It is also necessary to know the exact relationship between individuals as there may be confusion about the correct terminology (see Figures 13.4–13.7.

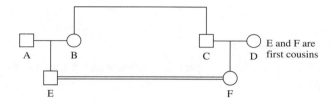

Figure 13.4 Marriage between First Cousins

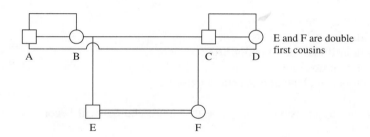

Figure 13.5 Marriage between Double First Cousins

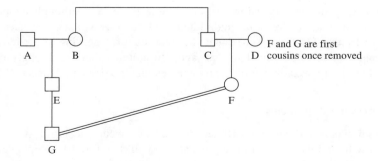

Figure 13.6 Marriage between First Cousins Once Removed

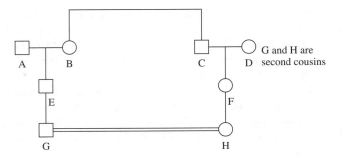

Figure 13.7 Marriage between Second Cousins

REPRODUCTIVE CHOICES

In Chapter 5, the choices that couples face when making reproductive decisions were explored:

- Avoid further pregnancies.
- Plan further pregnancies.

  1. accepting the risk
  2. with prenatal diagnosis
  3. with artificial insemination from a donor
  4. with egg donation
  5. with pre-implantation genetic diagnosis.

- Postpone the decision in the hope that more choices will become available in the near future.

Avoid Further Pregnancies

This is a very difficult decision for any couple to make. Although adoption is a possible alternative, for some individuals/cultures this will not be acceptable. Schott & Henley (1996, p. 188) state: 'In some cultures proving one's fertility is traditionally more important than marriage.' In cultures that are strongly centred around the family, avoiding further pregnancies may be deemed unacceptable.

Plan Further Pregnancies

Some individuals and cultures will accept whatever occurs, seeing it as God's (or a god's) will, and the risk in future pregnancies will therefore be acceptable.

However, others may wish to pursue the options of prenatal diagnosis, artificial insemination by donor (AID), egg donation or pre-implantation diagnosis. The majority of couples requesting prenatal diagnosis do so with the intention of terminating the pregnancy if the foetus is found to be affected with the genetic condition. However, termination of pregnancy (TOP) is not acceptable in all religions, and nor is assisted conception:

- Christianity: Varies according to denomination. For Roman Catholics, TOP is not acceptable under any circumstance, and pre-implantation genetic diagnosis may be rejected because of concerns about the unused embryos. Other creeds allow more personal choice.
- Hinduism: TOP is traditionally disapproved of but individual attitudes may vary.
- Islam: Many Muslims believe that TOP is forbidden, but there is some controversy regarding this. When a service for the prenatal diagnosis of beta-thalassaemia was introduced in Pakistan, two renowned Islamic scholars ruled that a pregnancy could be terminated if the foetus was affected by a serious genetic disorder and at less than 120 days' gestation (Ahmed et al., 2000). If the couple is unsure of what is acceptable, they should be advised to consult with their local Imam. AID and egg donation are not usually acceptable.
- Judaism: Orthodox Jews are unlikely to terminate a pregnancy, even when foetal abnormality is detected. AID and egg donation are not usually acceptable.
- Jehovah's Witnesses: TOP is not acceptable under any circumstances. AID and egg donation are not usually acceptable but decisions about pre-implantation genetic diagnosis will be left to the individual.
- Rastafarianism: TOP is traditionally disapproved of but individual attitudes may vary.
- Sikhism: TOP is traditionally disapproved of but individual attitudes may vary.

However, as previously mentioned, religious beliefs and personal practice are not always the same.

POST MORTEMS

- Christianity: No religious prohibition.
- Hinduism: Post mortem is not generally approved of but individuals may agree if the need is carefully explained.
- Islam: Post mortem is forbidden and most families are unlikely to agree.
- Judaism: Orthodox Jews are unlikely to agree to post mortem.
- Jehovah's Witnesses: No religious prohibition.
- Rastafarian: Post mortem is likely to be unacceptable.
- Sikhism: No religious prohibition.

When a post mortem cannot be conducted, other useful information may be obtained from photographs, X-rays, ultrasound and MRI scans, as well as from any DNA that may have been obtained prior to death.

INCIDENCE OF GENETIC DISORDERS AMONG DIFFERENT ETHNIC GROUPS

There is a link between certain recessive disorders and certain ethnic groups (Table 13.1). However, it is important to realise that although these disorders are more common within these ethnic groups, they are not confined to them. Inter-ethnic unions are common and result in gene mutations being more widely dispersed throughout the world population, and this must be remembered when considering national screening programmes.

Table 13.1 Link between Autosomal Recessive Disorders and Ethnic Groups

Ethnic Group	Disorder
Northern-European Caucasian	Cystic fibrosis
	Alpha 1-antitrypsin deficiency
	PKU
S. Asian and Mediterranean	Beta thalassaemia
	G6PD deficiency
	PKU
African	Sickle cell
African-Caribbean	G6PD deficiency
Ashkenazi Jewish	Tay Sachs disease
	Gaucher disease
	Cystic fibrosis
	Nonsyndromic hearing loss
	Canavan disease
	Familial dysautonomia
	Niemann-Pick disease
	Predisposition to breast cancer associated with the BRCA2 gene mutation (see Chapter 12)

It is suggested that some variations are due to the relative benefits conferred by carrier state in certain circumstances. For example, sickle cell disease is more common among African and African-Caribbean populations and beta thalassaemia is more common in the Mediterranean, the Middle East and Asia. Both these conditions give some protection against malaria, which was once very common in these areas but is less so now. Cystic fibrosis is more common among Northern-European Caucasians and is thought to have given protection against gastro-intestinal infections such as cholera and dysentery, and therefore to have been of some value several hundred years ago. Tay Sachs disease is more common amongst Askenazi Jews and is thought to give protection against tuberculosis.

CASE STUDY 1: TWO AUTOSOMAL RECESSIVE CONDITIONS IN THE SAME FAMILY

Abida and Tahir were referred to the clinical genetics unit following Abida's second miscarriage. Their first child had been born in Pakistan at 34 weeks' gestation.

The baby boy had multiple abnormalities and was not seen by either parent before his death at the age of nine hours. A post mortem had not been carried out and therefore no definitive information was available.

Abida and Tahir were seen by an Urdu speaking genetic counsellor as this was their first language. Tahir spoke English but Abida could not, although she understood some words. The family history revealed that they were double first cousins, as their fathers were brothers and their mothers were sisters.

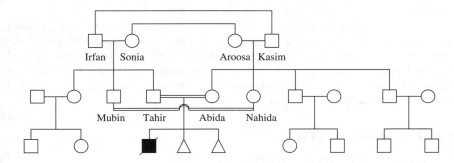

Pedigree 13.1

A history involving a child with multiple abnormalities and several miscarriages immediately arouses suspicion of a chromosome translocation inherited in an unbalanced form. As it was impossible to confirm this in Abida and Tahir's son, blood was taken from both parents to determine whether either of them carried a balanced chromosome translocation.

When the results were available, the couple was seen again to be told that they both had a normal chromosome pattern. They were advised that if their first child had had abnormal chromosomes, it was likely to be sporadic, with a very low risk of recurrence. However, as there was so little information, and Abida and Tahir were double first cousins, there was a possibility that their son had had an autosomal recessive condition, in which case there would be a 1 in 4 risk of recurrence. Although no diagnosis had been made, detailed scans could be offered in subsequent pregnancies.

Several months later, Abida contacted the genetic counsellor to tell her that she was pregnant. A detailed ultrasound scan was arranged at 18 weeks' gestation and did not reveal any structural abnormalities. The scan was repeated at 22 weeks for added reassurance and again no abnormalities were detected. Five months later, a very excited Abida contacted the genetic counsellor to tell her that she had delivered a little girl, Shabana, and all was well.

However, several weeks later Abida again contacted the genetic counsellor to tell her that neonatal screening had detected that Shabana had sensorineural deafness. Abida asked for a further appointment at the genetic clinic. Careful enquiries about Abida's health in the pregnancy had revealed no evidence of rubella or cytomegalovirus infection. Studies suggest that 40–50% of cases of sensorineural deafness are autosomal recessive (Harper, 2004, p. 260) and, given the degree of relationship between Abida and Tahir, this seemed the most likely cause in Shabana's case. Blood was taken from Shabana in order to look for alterations in the connexin 26 gene. Her parents were advised that a negative result would not exclude an autosomal recessive form of deafness as not all alterations are yet detectable. If the alterations were found then prenatal diagnosis would be available to the couple. Abida and Tahir made it clear that they would not wish to consider prenatal diagnosis as they would not contemplate terminating a pregnancy for this condition. In the event, no gene alterations were detected.

Abida and Tahir were understandably puzzled as to why they had not yet been able to have a healthy child. Although accepting the explanation of autosomal recessive inheritance, they also felt that it was the will of God and wondered what they had done to deserve this. These feelings were exacerbated when a year later, in the next pregnancy, a detailed scan showed that the foetus had features consistent with a diagnosis of Meckel syndrome.

Meckel Syndrome: The Disorder

This is an autosomal recessive condition characterised by:

- Encephalocele, in which the meninges herniate through the skull bones and may also contain brain tissue.
- Polycystic kidneys.
- Polydactyly, i.e. extra digits on the hands and/or feet.
- Cleft lip and palate.
- Eye defects.

The ultrasound scan showed a large encephalocele, polycystic kidneys and poly-dactyly. When Abida and Tahir realised the seriousness of the condition and the poor prognosis if the pregnancy continued to term, they consulted with their local Imam to determine whether termination of pregnancy would be acceptable. A decision was made, with great sadness, to terminate.

Following this, the genetic counsellor visited the family at their home to offer support and discuss the risks to future pregnancies. It was possible that this couple carried altered genes for two recessive conditions. Therefore, in each subsequent pregnancy there was a 1 in 4 risk for each of these conditions.

The couple was very pleased with Shabana's progress since she had been fitted with hearing aids. Although they would prefer to have a hearing child, they felt that Shabana's quality of life was good. However, they were very worried about the risk of another child with Meckel syndrome.

Counselling the Extended Family

Abida's sister, Nahida, was married to Tahir's brother, Mubin. Their other siblings were married to more distant relatives. Nahida and Mubin were therefore both at risk of being carriers for both conditions but did not want to be seen by the genetic counsellor as they had two healthy children and did not accept that there was a risk for them. The other siblings declined the offer of genetic counselling as there were no tests that could clarify their carrier status. Abida gave members of the extended family the name and contact number for the genetic counsellor in case they changed their minds.

Several months later, Nahida and Mubin contacted the genetic counsellor as Nahida was pregnant again and the couple was now anxious to clarify their situation. They didn't want their families to know that they were seeking advice and were reassured that their appointment would be confidential. The genetic counsellor was familiar with this request and with the fact that family members often only request genetic counselling when there is an ongoing pregnancy.

She explained autosomal recessive inheritance to Nahida and Mubin. Their actual carrier risk depended upon whether both sets of their parents (Irfan and Sonia, and Kasim and Aroosa) were carriers for either or both of the conditions.

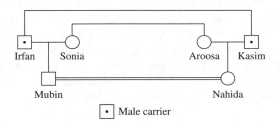

Pedigree 13.2

- If only one member of each set of parents (e.g. Irfan and Kasim or Sonia and Aroosa) was a carrier for congenital sensorineural deafness then Nahida and Mubin each had a 1 in 2 risk of being a carrier for the condition. The risk to each pregnancy would be: $1/2 \times 1/2 \times 1/4 = 1/16$.
- If all four of Nahida and Mubin's parents were carriers for congenital sensorineural deafness then Nahida and Mubin each had a 2 in 3 risk of being

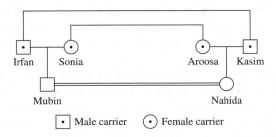

Pedigree 13.3

a carrier for the condition. The risk to each pregnancy would be: 2/3 X 2/3 X 1/4 = 4/36 = 1/9. The risk of having a child with Meckel syndrome would be the same.

Nahida and Mubin declined a detailed ultrasound scan as they felt they would not want to terminate a pregnancy. Although happy to comply with their wishes, the genetic counsellor was concerned that the couple still did not fully accept that there was a risk to their offspring because, unlike Abida and Tahir, they had already had two healthy children.

CASE STUDY 2: UNEXPECTED DIAGNOSIS WITHIN AN ETHNIC GROUP

David and Charlotte first became concerned about their second child, Henry, when he was seven months old. Up till then he had been a sociable little boy who was very responsive, sitting well unaided and grasping objects. They had first noticed that he was becoming less responsive and less interested in his feeds when he was six months old, but attributed this to teething as his older sister, Emily, had always been miserable when cutting teeth. However, they then noticed that Henry was becoming lethargic and floppy and no longer able to sit unaided. Henry was referred to a paediatrician by the family's general practitioner at the age of nine months and the diagnosis of Tay Sachs disease was made.

Tay Sachs: The Disorder

Tay Sachs is an autosomal recessive neuronal degenerative disorder. Affected infants usually present within the first six months of life, with a typical history of loss of response, poor feeding and floppiness. Loss of previously achieved milestones become apparent and the infant continues to deteriorate. Eventually they will become deaf and blind, and spastic paralysis of all four limbs will occur. They will usually die before the age of three.

Tay Sachs is a lysosomal storage disease. There is reduced activity of the enzyme hexosamidase A, which is required to break down fatty materials known as gangliosides, causing an abnormal build-up of a lipid GM2 ganglioside. The nerve cells in the brain are particularly affected. This condition is found most commonly in individuals of Ashkenazi Jewish ancestry, the carrier frequency in this population being 1 in 30.

David and Charlotte were devastated to discover that their son had a terminal illness. This was compounded when they realised that they must be carriers for the condition, as they felt that they had 'caused' it to happen. At this stage, Charlotte informed the paediatrician that she was pregnant and was horrified to be told that there was a 1 in 4 risk to this pregnancy. The couple was referred for an urgent genetic counselling appointment and was seen in the genetics clinic two days later.

Genetic Counselling

Charlotte and David were seen by a geneticist and genetic counsellor. They appeared very angry and hostile and found it difficult to accept the diagnosis and its implications for both Henry and the current pregnancy. This is a common response when an infant initially appears to be healthy and achieving developmental milestones, only to regress and be shown to have a degenerative condition which will lead to an early death.

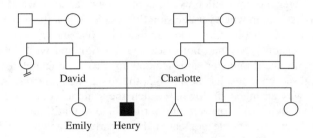

Pedigree 13.4

As expected, a family history revealed no previous indication of the condition in the family. Charlotte and David had been on the internet since receiving the diagnosis and were very angry to discover the association with Ashkenazi Jewish ancestry. They had traced their families back through several generations and found that they both came from well-established English ancestry with a strong Christian tradition. They also felt that there was little chance of them being evenly distantly related as Charlotte's family was from south-east England and David's family from Northumberland. The geneticist explained that although the disease was most commonly found among Ashkenazi Jewish families, it was not exclusive to that population.

Charlotte became very upset as she talked about her pregnancy, which was currently at eight weeks' gestation. The geneticist explained that it would be possible to offer prenatal diagnosis and the reason for the couple's hostility became apparent. Their strong religious belief had always led them to oppose termination of pregnancy for any reason. They had declined all screening tests in both previous pregnancies as they felt that they could cope with anything that could be wrong with a child. If they had considered the possibility of impairment at all, their thoughts had focused on Down syndrome. They felt that a child with Down syndrome would have the potential for a good quality of life and that they, as parents, could help to provide this.

They had been through agonies since Henry's diagnosis. They realised that not only would he die within the next few years, but that prior to his death he would cease to respond to them and his quality of life would decrease drastically. They did not feel that they could contemplate having another affected child, not only for the child's sake but also because of the effect on their daughter Emily, themselves, members of their extended family and their friends.

They were torn between their long-held beliefs about termination of pregnancy and the prospect of having another child with the disorder and all that that entailed. They needed to know if there was any way of avoiding an affected child in a future pregnancy. AID and egg donation were discussed but neither option was acceptable to the couple.

Charlotte and David were advised to give the matter further thought and it was agreed that the genetic counsellor would contact them again a week later to offer support and assistance in whatever decision they made. When the genetic counsellor next spoke with the couple, they told her that they had had a very difficult time coming to a decision. They had not discussed the situation with their family but had spoken with their minister and decided to have a prenatal test. CVS was carried out and sadly the results showed that the foetus was affected. A termination of pregnancy was arranged, following which the genetic counsellor again made contact, but the couple did not want any further help at that time.

Two years later, the couple contacted the department again as Charlotte was pregnant. Henry had died four months previously and it had been a time of great sadness for the family. Charlotte and David had decided to attempt one more pregnancy with prenatal diagnosis, as they hoped to have a healthy sibling for Emily.

They had also decided that whatever the results, Charlotte would request sterilisation, either following a termination or, hopefully, following the birth of an unaffected child. They did not feel that they could cope with the prospect of terminating more pregnancies after the current one. The genetic counsellor arranged the CVS and on this occasion the results were normal.

Throughout the interaction with this couple, the genetic counsellor was aware of hostility. This can happen when couples feel that circumstances have forced them to make decisions which they had previously thought unacceptable. Although the professionals involved had not applied pressure, leaving the couple to make their own decision, they had given the information that led to the choices the couple had to make. It is not unusual in this situation for a couple to feel angry towards the messenger. It is important for the professional not to react to this hostility but to accept that it is not personal and empathise with the couple's pain and anger. Clinical supervision is an excellent forum to discuss these issues and the feelings that they engender, allowing the healthcare professional to continue to work with the family and give support.

POINTS FOR REFLECTION

- How would you describe your culture?
- How aware are you of your own cultural assumptions and how they affect your understanding and responses?

- Culture is only one factor in an individual's life.
- Consider some of the benefits of other cultures as well as what you may perceive as disadvantages.
- Do you have regular clinical supervision?

REFERENCES

Ahmed, S. *et al.* (2000) Prenatal diagnosis of beta-thalassaemia in Pakistan: experience in a Muslim country. *Prenatal Diagnosis*, **20**(5), 378–83.

Bittles, A.H. (1998) *Empirical Estimates of the Global Prevalence of Consanguineous Marriage in Contemporary Societies*, Morrison Institute for Population and Resource Studies, Working Paper number 74, Stanford University, Stanford.

Culley, L. and Dyson, S. (2001) *Ethnicity and Nursing Practic.*, Palgrave, Basingstoke.

Harper, P.S. (2004) *Practical Genetic Counselling*, 6th edn, Arnold, London.

Ottenheimer, M. (1990) Lewis Henry Morgan and the prohibition of cousin marriage in the United States. *Journal of Family History*, **15**(3), 325–34.

Schott, J. and Henley, A. (1996) *Culture, Religion and Childbearing in a Multiracial Society*, Butterworth Heinemann, Oxford.

14 Ethical Issues

AMANDA BARRY

An individual's genetic information is extremely relevant to them personally, but the relevance to the individual's blood relatives and sexual partner should not be underestimated. Thus genetic information is generally seen as being family-centred and the value of sharing information within the family is recognised. But conflicts of interest do occur and they present ongoing ethical challenges to all professionals working in the field of clinical genetics. A case study will be used to illustrate the value of ethical theory and principles when developing strategies to inform and/or support decision making in such situations.

Further case studies will be used to encourage the reader to adopt a problem-solving approach to issues that include sharing of genetic information, testing of children, predictive testing for late-onset disorders and non-paternity.

The final section will consider issues such as discrimination, insurance, research and over-the-counter genetic tests from both an individual and a societal perspective.

PROFESSIONAL/PATIENT RELATIONSHIPS

Professional/patient relationships are based on respect for autonomy, privacy and maintenance of confidentiality. In particular, the patient's belief that information divulged will remain secret within the therapeutic environment underpins the relationship. Any actions which undermine this belief are likely to have repercussions for the individual, for the family and for society as a whole.

Ethical dilemmas arise in all clinical practice but the familial nature of genetics may lead to the belief that genetic ethical issues are inherently different. However, many argue that, while genetic information adds an extra dimension to these dilemmas, the basic situations are not unique to genetics. For instance, if an individual has a highly contagious illness, this must have relevance to those in contact with him and so sharing of the information could be deemed a moral, if not a legal, obligation.

In clinical practice, reference is made to the accepted ethical principles which underpin general medical practice when resolving difficult issues. There may well

Genetics in Practice: A clinical approach for healthcare practitioners   Edited by Jo Haydon
© 2007 John Wiley & Sons, Ltd

be occasions when an individual cannot be viewed in isolation and the interests of others must be considered paramount. Some dilemmas will remain unresolved in both general medical and genetic practice, and such cases require a decision tailored to the unique facts of the situation.

Sommerville & English suggest that, while the ethical dilemmas in genetics are not new, they have extra significance because of the family implications (Sommerville & English, 1999, p. 144). The Royal College of Physicians also concludes that the ethical problems of clinical genetics are of the same type as those in other areas of medicine, but recognises that questions have an added nuance because of the genetic basis of the conditions (Royal College of Physicians, 1991, p. 3). Many prestigious groups note that sharing of genetic information is not without risk. For instance, the Science and Technology Committee points out the possibility that uncontrolled distribution of genetic information could lead to discrimination (Science & Technology Committee, 1995, para. 225).

ETHICAL THEORY AND IMPLICATIONS FOR GENETICS

No one ethical theory can satisfactorily resolve all the varied clinical dilemmas faced by health professionals. Appeal to several different theories can provide greater insight and facilitate resolution. This can be illustrated in the following case study, about a family known to be at risk of the autosomal dominant condition Huntington disease (HD).

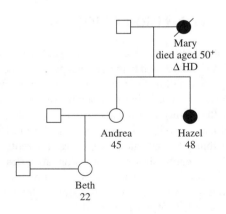

Pedigree 14.1

The maternal grandmother, Mary, died of HD in her early 50s, before any of her grandchildren were born. Her daughter, Andrea, aged 45 and symptomless, has a 1 in 2 (50%) risk of developing HD and investigated the possibility of having a predictive test but decided that she would prefer to leave things as they were. Her daughter, Beth, aged 22, had recently married and hoped to start a family in the near future. She had no knowledge of the family history. Beth consulted her GP for pre-conceptual advice. The GP had known the family for over 20 years and looked after Beth's affected aunt, Hazel, with whom Beth had no contact. The GP was therefore faced with an ethical dilemma as to what he should say to Beth.

ETHICAL PERSPECTIVES

From a **consequentialist perspective**, the GP could argue that he should act in such a way as to confer maximum benefit for all those concerned. This might lead him to decide that disclosing the family history would allow Beth and her partner to make an informed choice with regard to Beth's own risk and that of their planned child. He could also argue that the potential harm to Beth, her partner and their planned child was likely to be far greater than that to Andrea, who had been able to make an autonomous decision as to how she wished to cope with her risk of HD. Conversely, the GP might consider that the disruption caused to the family and to the GP's relationship with the family would outweigh the benefit to Beth.

Whose benefit should be paramount and how should the GP weigh up the conflicting benefits and harms to the different individuals? He should also be mindful of the possible repercussions for society if confidentiality were broken.

It can be argued that the GP owes a duty of care to both Andrea and Beth, as they are both his patients. His dilemma therefore is to try to ensure maximum benefit for both Andrea and Beth. Approaching Andrea in a non-specific way to suggest informing Beth of the family condition might be the best option. If Andrea were to decline, the GP would need to reconsider his duty to Beth, though making the decision to disclose against the wishes of Andrea would be difficult.

If viewed from a **deontological perspective**, the GP's prime duty is to Beth, since it is Beth who is making the specific enquiry. Deontological theory requires that each individual be treated as an end and not a means to an end, which supports Beth's right to the information she has requested. Genetic information is not just relevant to one individual, but to that individual's family. One could therefore argue that sharing such information is a duty, since the moral right of each family member must be respected. The GP might investigate other means of ensuring that Beth is informed of her risk, e.g. by suggesting to Andrea that Beth should be informed. Deontological theory emphasises the duty to the individual but as a result tends to ignore the interests of others. This is a problem when translating theory into practice.

If the GP considers a **rights-based approach**, informing Beth of the family history would be the only way of allowing Beth an informed autonomous choice. The competing rights of Andrea could be viewed as secondary to those of Beth. But equally, Andrea's right to confidentiality might be deemed to be as significant as Beth's right to make autonomous choices.

The GP could also consider the situation from a **communitarian perspective**, which recognises the responsibility of the community to the individual and the responsibility of the individual to the community. The GP might consider that his prime responsibility is to the common good, in this case the family good. The GP might therefore view Andrea's refusal to disclose the information to Beth as reprehensible and feel it is his duty to disclose the information.

Deontological and rights-based theories seem to favour the individual, Beth, whereas the consequentialist and communitarian theories emphasise the well-being of the family. Each of the four theories discussed encompass one overriding and absolute principle which must be adhered to. Such absolutist principles fail to address the conflicting rights encountered in clinical practice and therefore a less prescriptive approach may prove more effective.

BIOMEDICAL ETHICAL PRINCIPLES

Beauchamp & Childress have defined four basic principles suitable for biomedical practice, which are less rigid than the theories outlined above. The four principles are respect for autonomy, beneficence, non-maleficence and justice (Beauchamp & Childress, 1994, pp. 37–8).

Beauchamp & Childress state that the principles were initially derived from considered judgements in common morality and medical tradition. They describe them as 'general guides that leave considerable room for judgement in specific cases and that provide substantive guidance for the development of more detailed rules and policies' (Beauchamp & Childress, 1994, p. 38). The principles are considered to be obligations, defined as 'an obligation that must be fulfilled unless it conflicts on a particular occasion with an equal or stronger obligation' (Beauchamp & Childress, 1994, p. 33).

Respect for Autonomy

Current clinical practice, including that of the genetics service, and ethical discourse place great emphasis on respect for individual autonomy. Respect for autonomy recognises that an individual has the right of self-determination. Health professionals are well aware that given equivalent situations and identical information, different individuals will make different decisions. All individuals have varied life experiences, characteristics, values and beliefs, and thus decisions can only be made in the context of their personal lives (Lucassen & Rose, 1999, p. 314). This is a powerful argument for the nondirective and supportive ethos of the genetics service.

Autonomy is summarised by Gillon as 'The capacity to think, decide and act on the basis of such thought and decision freely and without let or hindrance' (Gillon, 1997, p. 60). An individual can only exercise their autonomy if other individuals and society as a whole respect their right to autonomy. This requires both respectful attitudes and respectful actions (Beauchamp & Childress, 1994, p. 125). The genetics service seeks to fulfil these requirements by providing information and support to those affected by or at risk of genetic conditions and thus enabling them to make their own decisions.

Harris goes further and argues that respecting the wishes of others acknowledges the value of the individual life. He states that 'Unless the value of our lives is to be undermined, the only constraint on our freedom to do as we please should be the familiar proviso that what we please to do does not harm others or does as little harm to others as it is possible for us to do' (Harris, 1985, p. 194).

Consideration of everyday life suggests that this is a persuasive argument, as individuals demonstrably value the right to make their own choices and rebel against constraints which they consider unjustified. Consequentialist and deontological moral theories support the individual's right to autonomy, though for very different reasons.

Beauchamp & Childress state that respect for autonomy does not overrule the obligation of others to try to dissuade individuals from taking ill-considered actions (Beauchamp & Childress, 1994, p. 125). Consider the HD family and the GP's dilemma again. If Andrea is showing early signs of HD, there is a possibility that her decisions are affected by reduced cognitive ability. Equally, Andrea's decision could be affected by erroneous information. For example, in this family only females have been affected so far and there may be a belief that all females will be affected and males unaffected. The GP has an obligation to make sure Andrea's decision is made with full knowledge of the facts and without impaired mental faculties.

An individual's autonomous actions might be considered unethical if they do serious harm to others. Whether the potential harm that could occur with regard to Beth is sufficiently serious to call Andrea's decision unethical is a contentious matter and one that would require further exploration. If Andrea had always hidden her diagnosis but was now so severely affected as to be unable to change the situation, the GP might decide that breaching her confidentiality could be justified.

There is no legal compulsion to inform Beth. Montgomery states that English law is reluctant to force people to assist one another (Montgomery, 1997, p. 263). He argues that this situation is not one where serious harm will be caused, but rather that Beth is being denied the opportunity of benefiting from the information. Others might consider that such a distinction is irrelevant as Beth is being denied the opportunity to take steps to avoid potential harm, at least to her offspring and partner.

Beneficence

Gillon describes beneficence as 'doing good for others', and he relates beneficence to the often-heard maxim of medical ethics: 'the patient's interests always come first'. He then points out that this would be an undesirable moral imperative and indeed can be demonstrated not to be one in medical practice (Montgomery, 1997, p. 263).

According to Beauchamp & Childress, 'the principle of beneficence refers to a moral obligation to act for the benefit of others' and is a positive requirement of particular relevance when some special relationship exists. They suggest that the principle is primary and therefore should be adhered to unless conflicting primary principles take precedence (Beauchamp & Childress, 1994, p. 260). They also point out that while the ideal of beneficence might suggest severe sacrifice, such sacrifice would not be obligatory as it could impose an impossible task. Further, they argue that the balancing of the costs and benefits which result from therapeutic actions is central to medical ethics. Thus actions that provide a benefit are often accompanied by a risk of harm. One could argue that this reinforces the importance of respect for an individual's autonomy as they should be able to decide whether to accept a risk given the probable benefit. In reconsidering the GP's dilemma, the principle of beneficence provides a strong argument in favour of respecting Andrea's decision not to inform Beth of the family history. But the risk involved relates to Andrea and does not take into account the risks to Beth. Could Andrea or the GP, who have a special relationship with Beth, be expected to act beneficently towards Beth, and might or should this special relationship influence their final decision?

Beauchamp & Childress argue that a person has an obligation of beneficence towards another if the following conditions (which are considered here using the HD example) are satisfied:

- An individual is at risk of significant loss of or damage to life or health or some other major interest: There are no interventions which can change the outcome for Beth if she has inherited the gene expansion which will lead to her developing HD. However, knowledge of her risk will allow Beth to make life decisions based on full information and thus it could be argued that Beth fulfils this criterion.
- Action is needed to prevent this loss or damage: Andrea would need to inform Beth herself or give permission for her GP to do so, or her GP would need to make the decision to inform Beth against Andrea's wishes.
- Action has a high probability of preventing the harm: This is more difficult to decide as informing Beth cannot prevent her inheriting HD, it can only allow her to make an autonomous decision with regard to the management of her risk. If Beth should be found to have inherited the gene for HD, there is no cure for the condition.
- Action would not present significant risks, costs or burdens to the individual: This is also difficult to assess as Andrea could well suffer harm as a result of disclosing the information about the family history and could feel pressured to reverse her previous decision with regard to predictive testing.
- The benefit that could be gained outweighs any harms, costs or burdens that might result: Once again this is difficult to assess as Beth may be caused considerable and enduring psychological harm by the new knowledge. If Beth resents receiving the knowledge, the effect on Andrea could be devastating.

Beauchamp & Childress point out that given the conditions above, conferring an obligation of beneficence on one person to benefit another is fraught with difficulty (Beauchamp & Childress, 1994, p. 266). The special relationship, primarily between

Andrea and Beth but also between the GP and Andrea and the GP and Beth, makes the situation even more problematic.

Non-maleficence

Gillon suggests that the scope of the principle of non-maleficence, 'avoidance of doing harm', is general and encompasses everyone. However, he disagrees with some writers who suggest that the principle of non-maleficence should take precedence over all others and argues that this would be unsustainable (Gillon, 1997, p. 81). He states that this is particularly the case in clinical practice, as often the action taken in the spirit of beneficence also carries the risk of harm.

Beauchamp & Childress agree that giving precedence to the principle of non-maleficence is not justifiable as the merit of other moral principles varies according to the circumstances and should be considered for each situation. They point out that the rule of non-maleficence requires avoidance of actions that cause harm, whereas the rules of beneficence relate to taking actions to help others (Beauchamp & Childress, 1994, pp. 191–2). This appears to be a reasonable distinction, but what of our GP who is trying to avoid harm and do good for both his patients, Andrea & Beth?

Justice

Beauchamp & Childress describe justice as a group of norms for distributing benefits, risks and costs (Beauchamp & Childress, 1994, p. 38). There are many theories of justice, which will not be discussed in depth here. Beauchamp & Childress state that there is a minimum requirement in all theories of justice, which can be attributed to Aristotle: 'Equals must be treated equally, and unequals must be treated unequally' (Beauchamp & Childress, 1994, p. 328). This means that if several individuals find themselves in equivalent situations, each should be treated equally with the other. If, however, their situations are dissimilar in any way, then this can result in one individual being deemed to have a greater claim.

Consider our HD family again. Suppose Beth had an identical twin sister, Claire, and they were both aware of the diagnosis in their maternal grandmother. If both Beth and Claire were newly married and wanting to start families, they should be treated equally. This would be relatively easy if both wished to act in the same way. However, if Beth wished to pursue predictive testing and Claire did not, the professionals involved would face a difficult dilemma. As Beth and Claire are identical twins, the predictive test on Beth would also disclose Claire's status. So if Beth was tested, she would have information about Claire which Claire had specifically stated she did not want to know. Beth might decide to keep her decision to opt for predictive testing secret in order to respect her sister's informed choice not to know. While this may seem a viable option, in practical terms it is likely to put a strain on the sisters' relationship whatever the outcome. How should the professionals proceed and whose rights would be considered paramount?

The four biomedical ethical principles discussed underpin the GP's deliberations as he endeavours to reach a decision that takes into account the wishes and rights of all those involved. The thought experiments serve to show that there is no easy answer to any dilemma in which there is a conflict of interest. Careful consideration of all the consequences of any decision is essential to the well-being of the individual, the family and society as a whole. Even when justifiable, the disclosure of information against an individual's wishes is a very grave step indeed.

ETHICAL DILEMMAS IN GENETIC PRACTICE

In order to make difficult choices, individuals need access to genetic counselling that provides accurate and understandable information about the condition, their risks and options. When referred for genetic counselling, an individual's expectations of the service they are accessing may be minimal or unrealistic. In some cases they may be unaware of or have misunderstand why they have been referred. Such issues need to be addressed before effective counselling can occur. The professionals concerned should also be aware of the need to discuss the implications for the extended family if a genetic basis for the condition is confirmed.

Every effort should be made to ensure that the relationship between doctor (or other health professional) and patient is a mutually effectual one. This relationship is of particular importance because the patient may have to relinquish (at least in the short term) their physical and/or psychological well-being to their carer. A good relationship underpinned by trust will allow the patient to interact with professionals without constraint and promote compliance with investigations and treatment. Inherent in the relationship is respect for an individual's autonomy, privacy and confidentiality. Such relationships are founded not just on individual trust, but also on the trust felt by society in general towards the medical and related professions. Actions that undermine the relationship could result in individuals and families deciding either not to seek out or not to accept the information/treatment they require.

CASE STUDY 1: SHARING GENETIC INFORMATION

Alan, aged 20, collapsed and was admitted to hospital, where he was found to be extremely anaemic. Further investigations showed that bleeding from bowel polyps had caused his anaemia. A diagnosis of familial adenomatous polyposis coli (FAP) was made.

Neither Alan nor his younger sister, Bethan, had been aware that the bowel cancer that caused their mother's death some years previously was the result of a genetic condition. Alan and Bethan were very close and he was keen to ensure that she received all the relevant information and to support her in any interventions aimed at managing her risk. The situation was different with regard to his aunt, Dawn, with whom he no longer spoke. The geneticist was particularly concerned about Dawn as she was older and therefore at greater risk.

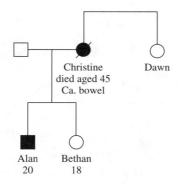

Pedigree 14.2

Ethical Issues

- What are the geneticist's responsibilities with regard to Dawn?
- Would you consider that Alan had a responsibility with regard to Dawn and if so, why?
- How might these responsibilities be met if Alan does not wish to have contact with Dawn?

As Dawn is not the geneticist's patient, the geneticist cannot be said to owe Dawn a duty of care. However, because the family is seen as central to genetic practice she does have a responsibility to highlight Dawn's risk to Alan and ensure that he understands the possible implications of not informing Dawn of this risk. If Alan declines, the geneticist is unlikely to be able to contact Dawn unless Alan discloses the demographic information required to do so.

But does Alan have a duty of care to Dawn because of their special relationship, i.e. being blood relatives? Some would argue that this is the case and indeed Alan has shown that he is willing to disclose the information to his sister. Certainly there is no legal duty on an individual to inform their relatives, but there can be said to be a moral duty (British Medical Association, 1998, p. 71). Assuming that the family rift is extremely serious, Alan might argue that any perceived duty to Dawn is no longer relevant because of past experiences. Further discussion might result in a way forward being identified, for example, Alan giving permission for the geneticist to contact Dawn's GP.

CASE STUDY 2: TESTING OF CHILDREN

Consider again the family described in the previous case study.

Let us suppose that some years have passed and, following relevant treatment, Alan has married and had two children, now aged 8 and 10. He is re-referred to the genetics service as he wishes to discuss molecular testing for his children. Since the alteration in the APC gene is known, the test will be technically easy to perform.

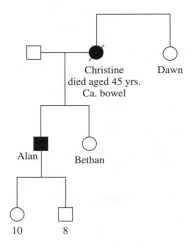

Pedigree 14.3

Ethical Issues

- Is such a test justifiable?
- What are the geneticist's responsibilities with regard to the children?

Given the children's ages, their ability to consent for themselves is likely to be limited. It could be argued that allowing the parents to request and consent to the genetic test ignores the children's future right as adults to make their own autonomous decisions, as well as their right to confidentiality. However, allowing the parents to request the test is considered justifiable in this situation as the bowel polyps start to appear from the teen years onwards and screening is generally commenced in the second decade. If one or both of the children is shown not to have inherited the mutation, they will not have to undergo screening, saving them the distress and anxiety which regular sigmoidoscopy/colonoscopy might cause. If one or both of the children is found to have inherited the mutation, the need for regular screening will be reinforced and the parents and child concerned will have time to consider and plan for their future surgical treatment. Thus the children's right to autonomy and confidentiality might be considered less important than the potential avoidance of harm and possible benefits outlined. The professionals involved will still endeavour to ensure that the children are included in the decision-making process and that the family is adequately prepared for all possible outcomes, including the possible implications if one child has inherited the gene and the other has not.

The testing of children may be justifiable in genetic conditions of early onset (e.g. FAP) or in conditions of late/sudden onset where treatment is available (e.g. familial hypercholesterolaemia or long QT syndrome). Each individual case will be considered on its own merits as it is important to recognise the possible adverse effects to children of knowing they have a genetic condition, such as stigmatisation, a blighted childhood and later problems with insurance and employment.

But what if the condition is of late onset and currently untreatable? The professionals concerned need to consider whether there are any benefits in proceeding with such a test. To whom do those benefits relate? The parents might argue that they need to know their child's status in order to plan for the future but is this truly a benefit for the child or might it actually be harmful to them, resulting in some form of discrimination? When the child becomes an adult they may regret the loss of confidentiality they have endured. They may wish they did not know their status, but the 'right not to know' will have been denied them. The parents' knowledge that their child has inherited the gene mutation and will be affected in later life could lead to overprotectiveness or restriction of the child's future life choices. Thus it is generally considered that unless there is a sound clinical reason for performing a test, children should not be tested until they are adults (Advisory Committee on Genetic Testing, 1998, p. 16; British Medical Association, 1998, pp. 89–93; World Health Organisation, 1997).

CASE STUDY 3: PREDICTIVE TESTING FOR LATE-ONSET DISORDERS

Predictive testing of adults for untreatable late-onset genetic conditions poses considerable challenges for genetic professionals. Adequate counselling is an essential prerequisite to such tests but can present unexpected situations.

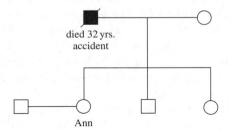

died 32 yrs.
accident

Ann

Pedigree 14.4

Ann was aware that her father had been diagnosed with myotonic dystrophy (MD) prior to his death, which was the result of an accident. His death predated Ann's marriage and she had never discussed the family history with her partner. Ann had not experienced any problems herself but was aware that she was at a 1 in 2 (50%) risk of having inherited the altered gene. She therefore requested a predictive test for MD.

Genetic Counselling

The inheritance of MD and the risk to any offspring were discussed and the geneticist asked if Ann's partner was aware of the situation. When told that he was not, the geneticist discussed the possible implications for their relationship of not telling him. The geneticist also discussed the implications for Ann of having a positive result. These included the possibility of anticipation (the phenomenon which results in an expansion of the gene mutation and thus the severity of the condition when the altered gene is passed from mother to child). A woman who has inherited the MD gene has a risk of having a baby with congenital MD. The size of the risk varies according to whether she is currently asymptomatic (less than 5%) or affected (10–30%), or has already had one affected child (40%). Babies with congenital MD have severe muscle weakness at birth, which can necessitate intensive respiratory support in the neonatal period and can prove fatal.

The geneticist felt that the woman's desire not to inform her partner at this stage should be respected and, after suitable counselling, proceeded with the test. The test result showed that Ann carried the altered form of the gene.

Ethical Issues

• What should the geneticist's response be if the woman still refuses to inform her partner at this stage?
• What about the rights of other family members, for instance Ann's siblings, who may be unaware of the family history?

It can be argued that Ann has a duty to inform both her partner and at-risk relatives because of their special relationship. The geneticist does not have the same duty of care to Ann's partner and relatives as he does to Ann. However, the family is seen as central to the genetics service so in practice it is generally agreed that professionals should encourage individuals to inform their blood relatives and partners (Genetic Interest Group, 1998, p. 10; Nuffield Council on Bioethics, 1993, p. 43).

If Ann refuses to disclose the relevant information to other at-risk relatives, the geneticist has to consider whether the harm that may result from their not being informed is sufficient to warrant disclosure without consent. Opinions regarding such disclosure are conflicting. The House of Commons Science & Technology Committee states that 'if counselling cannot persuade someone to consent to sharing information with their relatives the individual's decision to withhold information should be paramount' (Science & Technology Committee, 1995, para. 228). The Nuffield Council on Bioethics concluded that 'in exceptional circumstances, health professionals might be justified in disclosing genetic information to other family members despite an individual's desire for confidentiality' (Nuffield Council on Bioethics, 1993, para. 5.42). This type of dilemma can only be resolved by careful consideration of all the pertinent facts of the case. In practice, it may be impossible to contact at-risk individuals without Ann's cooperation in providing the relevant demographic information.

CASE STUDY 4: NON-PATERNITY

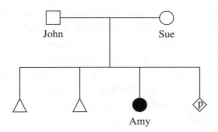

Pedigree 14.5

Sue and John had a child, Amy, who was recently diagnosed as having cystic fibrosis (CF). Sue was pregnant again and the couple was referred to the clinical genetic unit to discuss prenatal diagnosis. The couple was aware of the 1 in 4 (25%) risk of the baby inheriting CF and felt that a prenatal test was the only option for them. However, in view of Sue's previous history of miscarriages, both she and John were concerned about the risks associated with the prenatal diagnostic tests available to them (CVS or amniocentesis).

Blood specimens from both parents were obtained, as is normal practice, to confirm their carrier status and any CF alterations. The results showed that Sue was a carrier but that John was not. The results were checked and confirmed by the laboratory, suggesting that John was not Amy's biological father.

Ethical Issues

- How should the genetic professionals involved deal with this difficult situation?
- To whom and how should these results be disclosed?

Sue and John came to discuss the situation as a couple and thus the genetic professionals owe a duty of care to both of them. Both agreed to have blood tests and expect that their results will be available to them. The results would generally be given to the two of them together but could also be given individually. Research has shown that professionals faced with this sort of dilemma often choose to discuss the results with the mother first (Wertz & Fletcher, 1991, pp. 216–19) in the hope that this will cause the least harm to the couple, even though their actions could be seen as contrary to their duty of care to the man. Giving Sue the information first gives her the opportunity to clarify the situation. John may well be aware of the possibility that Amy is not his child and the couple may have chosen to ignore this possibility for their own reasons. If so, an open discussion with the couple would confirm non-paternity but would also reassure the couple that the baby they were expecting was not at risk of CF and that the miscarriage risk of prenatal testing (0.5–2%) could be avoided.

A much more difficult scenario will occur if John had no idea that there was a possibility that Amy might not be his child. John has a right to be given his results but by doing so, disclosure of non-paternity is inevitable. This would be likely to be detrimental to John's relationship with both Sue and Amy. What if Sue asks the geneticist to respect her need for confidentiality and not disclose the results, and to proceed with CVS as if both parents were carriers? If the geneticist agreed, he would be putting his duty of care to John and John's right to know second to the desire to avoid causing harm to the family as a whole. But what about the risk involved in conducting a prenatal test which is completely unnecessary? Can this additional risk be justified?

Such situations may be avoided by careful pre-test counselling but there will always be occasions when discussion is less than optimal. Once the situation has occurred there are no easy answers, but careful counselling may lead to an agreed resolution. However, some dilemmas cannot be satisfactorily resolved and this is when discussion with the genetics team is invaluable. While the final decision may need to be made by one or two professionals, they should never feel unsupported when doing so (Genetic Interest Group, 1998, p. 14).

GENETICS AND SOCIETY

In recent years the increasing emphasis upon individual as opposed to collective responsibility has resulted in increased applications for health, disability and mortgage protection plans (British Medical Association, 1998, p. 156). Individuals with adverse family histories or those at risk of genetic conditions are at a disadvantage when seeking such cover as they are charged greater premiums than other people. Insurance companies justify this situation by arguing that the premium should reflect risk. Ethically this can be justified, as 'Equals must be treated equally, and unequals must be treated unequally' (Beauchamp & Childress, 1994, p. 328).

This seems reasonable in cases where the individual had some control over the cause of their increased risk, for instance if they chose to smoke or to take part in hazardous sports. But increased risk as a result of family history or genetic conditions is outside the influence of the individual. It could be argued that everyone faces other, albeit small, risks that are outside their control, for instance of being injured as a result of freak weather conditions or as an innocent bystander. Also, we are all at risk of becoming unexpectedly ill at some point in our lives.

Is it discriminatory to load premiums for individuals with genetic conditions, especially since it might mean they are unable to afford insurance? An alternative would be to spread the increased risk of the minority by raising the premiums for all. The insurance companies deem this to be unfair to the majority, but the BMA suggests that this sort of collectivist position would reflect the insurance companies' social responsibilities (British Medical Association, 1998, p. 167). This is the subject of much debate between all interested parties. One aim is to ensure that individuals at risk of genetic conditions do not find themselves in a situation whereby they cannot access insurance. Equally, it is essential to ensure that the burden on the majority who are not at risk is not so onerous as to reduce their willingness to take out adequate insurance.

It is recognised that mandatory genetic testing in order to determine insurance premiums would unfairly discriminate against those with a family history of a genetic condition. Such compulsion would effectively compromise the individual's right to autonomy and could easily cause actual harm in the form of psychological sequelae resulting from the test being agreed to under duress. A positive result could also lead to difficulties with employment and career progression. There is concern that if individuals were compelled to disclose the results of any genetic tests, people would be less likely to request testing. This could result in lost opportunities with regard to surveillance, prophylactic or active treatments and prenatal diagnosis.

While non-consensual disclosure of genetic information to insurance companies is not justifiable, it could be argued that on occasion society's knowledge of an individual's genetic makeup could be beneficial. For example, the BMA highlights the advantage of improved access to services such as special needs education and social service support (British Medical Association, 1998, p. 153). Despite this, there are many other instances when an individual could be disadvantaged, pressured or even discriminated against as a result of information about them being known. Kitcher argues that 'Individual choices are not made in a social vacuum, and unless changes in social attitudes keep pace with the proliferation of genetic tests, we can anticipate that many future prospective parents, acting to avoid misery for potential children, will have to bow to social attitudes they reject and resent' (Kitcher, 1997, p. 199).

Garver & Garver state that when the option of prenatal diagnosis was introduced into medical practice it was based within the patient/doctor relationship. They go on to register their concern that in the future prenatal diagnosis could become public policy and that as a result, individual patients might lose the right to make their own decisions (Garver & Garver, 1991, p. 1115). For instance, society might develop the view that the individual is acting irresponsibly if they fail to take advantage of the offer of prenatal diagnosis or if they decide not to terminate an affected foetus. If this were to occur, it could be accompanied by the insidious withdrawal of services and support for those disadvantaged by their genetic blueprint or an accident of birth – a very chilling thought!

Some writers, particularly groups representing those with disabilities, express concern about the marginalisation and stigmatisation of those deemed not to be 'normal' (Nuffield Trust, 2000, p. 25). When considering these concerns, Morgan argues that the offer of prenatal diagnosis does not necessarily imply that a woman, a couple or the health service believes that people with handicaps are less 'entitled to life' than people without handicaps (Morgan, 1996, p. 200). He points out that this belief could disguise a gradual shift towards more eugenic policies. Pembrey argues convincingly that 'the goal of genetic and prenatal diagnostic provision must be to help these couples make an informed choice, one which they feel is best for themselves and their families' (Pembrey, 1991, p. 1267).

But what if the state were to decide that it was necessary to intervene? Garver & Garver refer to several writers who, when considering the high cost of medical care in the USA, have suggested that a reduction in healthcare for newborns with congenital or genetic disease, and for elderly people who are incompetent or chronically ill, could be an acceptable way of making savings (Garver & Garver, 1991, p. 1115). We might believe that the eugenic policies of the past will never be allowed to occur again but this seems both naïve and irrelevant as the lay public and professionals alike remain concerned about this possibility (Boddington, 1994, pp. 224, 239; McLean, 2000, p. 3; Nuffield Trust, 2000, p. 25). Respect for autonomy and privacy remains vital and any decisions made by individuals should not be subject to coercion from any source.

There are legitimate reasons for supporting genetic research, and for this to be effective we need the cooperation of those families affected by genetic conditions. Cooperation could easily be withdrawn if the individuals concerned were worried that their right to confidentiality and privacy was being ignored. This would be to the detriment of all concerned, since research into one condition can have relevance to others. Who knows what genes have been inherited or what new alterations have occurred during meiosis? Any one of us could succumb to a genetic disorder that we are currently unaware of having. The need for the full and informed consent of all individuals who agree to participate in research and for the safeguards provided by research ethics committees are generally accepted and will not be discussed further here (British Medical Association, 1998, p. 137; Montgomery, 1997, p. 338; Nuffield Trust, 2000, pp. 38–9).

More and more genetic tests are now available, some of them over the counter. The BMA notes the unease felt by many who are concerned that the companies offering this type of service are not able to ensure that clients understand the implications of the tests, or to provide access to appropriate counselling, thus compromising the individual's ability to make a truly informed choice (British Medical Association, 1998, p. 113). In 1997, the then Advisory Committee on Genetic Testing (ACGT) developed a voluntary code of practice under which companies were expected to submit their proposals. The ACGT published an annual report, which listed those companies that adhered to the code. The code restricted screening for carrier status of recessive conditions where there were no significant health implications for the individual. Those under 16 and adults without the capacity to consent were not to be screened. Individuals with a family history of genetic disorder were to be advised to seek testing through a medical practitioner (Advisory Committee on Genetic Testing, 1998). The Human Genetics Commission (HGC) has since extended the code to include paternity testing (Human Genetics Condition, 2002).

The Human Genetics Commission was set up in 1999 when, after a comprehensive review, it was recommended that, while the regulatory systems were working well, the advisory framework needed to:

- Be more transparent, in order to gain public and professional confidence.
- Be more streamlined, in order to avoid gaps, overlaps and fragmentation.
- Ensure capacity to deal with rapid developments and to take broad social and ethical issues fully into account.

Since its formation, the HGC has endeavoured to consult widely and, in particular, to engage with the general public. Giving the public the opportunity to understand ethical dilemmas in genetics and to influence possible guidelines for practice seems to be a good way of ensuring that patient/professional relationships are not adversely affected by misunderstanding and scepticism. Decisions made now will influence the future, and it is the future use of genetic information which most concerns the individual, their family and society as a whole.

POINTS FOR REFLECTION

* Ethical dilemmas such as those highlighted in the case studies emphasise the importance of an effective professional relationship with the patient, which is built on mutual respect and trust.
* Working with the patient and their family is the most effective way to bring about satisfactory resolution of conflicts of interest.
* The family focus of the genetics service gives added nuances to ethical dilemmas.
* Can you think of any ethical dilemmas related to genetics where breach of confidentiality could be justified that might occur in your own practice? If so, how would you deal with the situation?

REFERENCES

Advisory Committee on Genetic Testing (1998) *Genetic Testing for Late Onset Disorders*, Health Departments of the United Kingdom, London.

Beauchamp, T. and Childress, J. (1994) *Principles of Biomedical Ethics*, Oxford University Press, New York.

Boddington, P. (1994) Confidentiality in genetic counselling. In: *Genetic Counselling: Practice and Principles* (ed. Clarke, A.), Routledge, London.

British Medical Association (1998) *Human Genetics: Choice and Responsibility*, Oxford University Press, London.

Garver, K. and Garver, B. (1991) Eugenics: Past, present and the future. *American Journal of Human Genetics*, **49**, 1109–18.

Genetic Interest Group (1998) *Confidentiality Guidelines*, Genetic Interest Group, London.

Gillon, R. (1997) *Philosophical Medical Ethics*, J. Wiley & Sons, Chichester.

Harris, J. (1985) *The Value of Life*, Routledge, London.

Human Genetics Commission (2002) Available at: www.hgc.gov.uk.

Kitcher, P. (1997) *The Lives to Come*, Penguin, London.

Lucassen, A. and Rose, P. (1999) *Practical Genetics for Primary Care*, Oxford University Press, Oxford.

McLean, S. (2000) International justice: A brave new world or a leap in the dark. *Genetics Law*, **1**, 1–3.

Montgomery, J. (1997) *Health Care Law*, Oxford University Press, Oxford.

Morgan, D. (1996) The troubled helix: Legal aspects of the new genetics. In: *The Troubled Helix* (eds Marteau, T. and Richards, M.), Cambridge University Press, Cambridge.

Nuffield Council on Bioethics (1993) *Genetic Screening: Ethical Issues*, Nuffield Council on Bioethics, London.

Nuffield Trust, Genetics Scenario Project (2000) *Genetics and Health*, The Stationery Office, Norwich.

Pembrey, M. (1991) Letters to editor: Non-directive counselling. *The Lancet*, **338**, 1267.

Royal College of Physicians (1991) *Ethical Issues in Clinical Genetics*, Royal College of Physicians, London.

Science & Technology Committee (1995) Third report: Human genetics: The science and its consequences. HMSO, House of Commons, London.

Sommerville, A. and English, V. (1999) Genetic privacy: Orthodoxy or oxymoron? *Journal of Medical Genetics*, **25**, 144–50.

Wertz, D. and Fletcher, J. (1991) Privacy and disclosure in medical genetics examined in an ethics of care. *Bioethics*, **5**(3), 212–31.

World Health Organisation (1997) Proposed international guidelines on ethical issues in medical genetics and genetic services. Document reference: WHO/HGN/GL/ETH/98.1, No longer available online (Accessed 25/06/00).

15 Professional Development

AMANDA BARRY AND JO HAYDON

The first clinical genetic departments in the UK were set up in the 1950s. The need for, and value of, multidisciplinary input was recognised and led to the appointment of the first genetic nurse in 1959.

Currently there are 25 specialist clinical genetics departments in the United Kingdom. Most are co-located with, or have strong ties to, both service laboratories and university academic departments.

Clinical centres are staffed by medical geneticists, specialist genetic registrars and genetic counsellors, along with support staff such as medical secretaries, administrators and IT specialists. Some centres also have input from other professionals such as psychologists, ethicists, patient support group care advisors and Genetic Interest Group project workers.

Most centres cover a wide geographical region and therefore hold outreach clinics in various locations around their area. In recent years there has been a move towards genetic counsellors being based within the community they serve, e.g. in district general hospitals or primary care trusts. These developments seek to improve patients' access to the service and to raise awareness among health professionals and the families that might benefit.

This aim is even more important now that genetics is being recognised as affecting all aspects of health and disease. The specialist service will be required to support practitioners as they develop, extend and incorporate the necessary knowledge and skills to provide basic genetic information within primary care.

GENETIC COUNSELLING

The specialist genetic centres seek to ensure that the genetic counselling offered fulfils the aims of the following widely accepted definition, which states that genetic counselling is:

> a communication process which deals with human problems associated with the occurrence, or risk of occurrence, of a genetic disorder in a family. This process involves

Genetics in Practice: A clinical approach for healthcare practitioners   Edited by Jo Haydon
© 2007 John Wiley & Sons, Ltd

an attempt by one or more appropriately trained persons to help the individual or family to (1) comprehend the medical facts, including the diagnosis, probable course of the disorder and the available management (2) appreciate the way in which heredity contributes to the disorder and the risk of recurrence in specified relatives (3) understand the alternatives for dealing with the risk of recurrence (4) choose the course of action which seems to them appropriate in the view of their risk, their family goals and their ethical and religious standards and to act in accordance with that decision (5) and to make the best possible adjustment to the disorder in an affected family member and/or to the risk of recurrence of that disorder (American Society of Human Genetics, 1975).

Within the specialist centres, the genetic counselling team comprises medical and non-medical professionals responsible for the process of genetic counselling.

MEDICAL GENETICISTS

Medical geneticists include consultant geneticists, specialist genetic registrars and in some units psychiatrists and hospital practitioners. Medical doctors are able to train as clinical geneticists after a suitable period of postgraduate experience. Medical geneticists will have previously specialised in one of a variety of specialties, including general medicine, paediatrics and neurology.

GENETIC COUNSELLORS

In the early days of the profession, most genetic counsellors came from a nursing, midwifery or health visiting background, with a small number coming from social work. Since 1992 it has been possible to enter the profession via an approved master's degree in genetic counselling.

There is a clear difference between those genetic counsellors who work with families at high genetic risk and those professionals who require basic genetic knowledge to underpin their own roles, for instance professionals working in family history clinics, infertility clinics or haematology (Association of Genetic Nurses and Counsellors, 2003).

ASSOCIATION OF GENETIC NURSES AND COUNSELLORS (AGNC)

By the late 1970s there were approximately 30 nurses, health visitors and social workers working in clinical genetics departments. Most were the only non-medical genetic professional in their department and were therefore isolated from their peers. In 1980, the need to establish better professional links led to a meeting which resulted in the formation of the Genetic Nurses and Social Workers Association (GNSWA). The name of the association was changed in 1995 to the Association of Genetic Nurses and Counsellors (AGNC) in recognition of the growing number of members from a non-nursing/social work background.

When the association was first established, its aims were to:

- Help provide better standards of care for families through the exchange of ideas and information.
- Combat isolation for those working on their own.
- Establish appropriate education for members in clinical departments (Weetman, 2002).

These aims are still generally appropriate, although most genetic counsellors no longer work in isolation.

From an early stage, the association forged links with the Clinical Genetics Society (CGS) and, along with the CGS, became one of the founder groups of the British Society of Human Genetics (BSHG) in 1996. The BSHG is able to provide a united response regarding genetic issues, an important role of considerable benefit when negotiating genetic contracts nationally. The constituent groups (clinicians, cytogeneticists, molecular geneticists, cancer geneticists and genetic counsellors) still maintain their own separate professional identities.

In more recent years, various AGNC sub-committees have been set up with the aim of advancing the recognition of genetic counselling as a profession. Issues which have been addressed include voluntary (and potentially statutory) registration, career structure, safe and ethical practice, code of ethics (Box 15.1), education and supervision. The AGNC has accepted the working party recommendation that 'The term genetic counsellor is adopted in the United Kingdom as the title for non-medical health professionals working in clinical settings, providing genetic counselling' (Association of Genetic Nurses and Counsellors, 2003).

Box 15.1 AGNC Code of Ethics

Self awareness and development
Genetic counsellors should:

- Recognise the limits of their own knowledge and abilities in any given situation and decline any duties or responsibilities that cannot be carried out in a safe and competent manner.
- Be responsible for their own physical and emotional health as it impacts on their professional performance.
- Report to an appropriate person or authority any conscientious objection that may be relevant to their professional practice.
- Maintain and improve their own professional education and competence.

Box 15.1 (Continued)

Relationships with clients
Genetic counsellors should:

- Enable clients to make informed independent decisions, free from coercion.
- Respect the client's personal beliefs and their right to make their own decisions.
- Avoid any abuse of their professional relationship with clients.
- Protect all the confidential information concerning clients obtained in the course of professional practice: disclosures of such information should only be made with the client's consent, unless disclosure can be justified because of a significant risk to others.
- Report to an appropriate person or authority any circumstance, action or individual that may jeopardise client care, or their health and safety.
- Seek all relevant information required for any given client situation.
- Refer clients to other competent professionals if they have needs outside the professional expertise of the genetic counsellor.

Relationships with colleagues
Genetic counsellors should:

- Collaborate and co-operate with other colleagues in order to provide the highest quality of service to the client.
- Foster relationships with other members of the clinical genetics team, to ensure that clients benefit from a multidisciplinary approach to care.
- Assist colleagues to develop their knowledge of clinical genetics and genetic counselling.
- Report to an appropriate person or authority any circumstance or action which may jeopardise the health and safety of a colleague.

Responsibilities within the wider society
Genetic counsellors should:

- Provide reliable and expert information to the general public.
- Adhere to the laws and regulations of society. However, when such laws are in conflict with the principles of the profession, genetic counsellors should work toward change that will benefit the public interest.
- Seek to influence the policy makers on human genetic issues, both as an individual and through membership of professional bodies.

(Association of Genetic Nurses and Counsellors, 2000a)

QUALIFICATIONS REQUIRED PRIOR TO PRACTICE AS A GENETIC COUNSELLOR

In the past, experienced professionals from a nursing, midwifery or health visiting, and to a lesser extent from a scientific or social work background were appointed as 'co-workers' within specialist genetic departments. In general, each centre was autonomous and therefore both local service provision and the expectations of the co-worker role developed in a very ad hoc fashion. This resulted in a plethora of titles and variability in practice. As the discipline developed it became increasingly obvious that:

- The different modes of entry into the genetic counsellor role did not fit easily within any one professional body.
- More formal training was required to prepare individuals for the role.
- Experienced practitioners were extending their role to include increasingly autonomous practice such as adopting specialised roles and taking responsibility for a locally determined range of non-diagnostic consultations.

An education working party was convened to determine the needs of the emerging profession and, in particular, the way forward with regard to becoming a self-regulating and inclusive profession. The AGNC membership approved the recommendations of the working party in 2000 by adopting a competency-based, voluntary assessment process for registration as a genetic counsellor.

Box 15.2 AGNC Core Competencies

Client/counsellor relationship

- Establish relationship and elicit client's concerns and expectations.
- Elicit and interpret appropriate medical, family and psychological history.
- Convey clinical and genetic information to clients appropriate to their individual needs.
- Explain options available to the client, including risks, benefits and limitations.
- Acknowledge the implications of individual and family experiences, beliefs, values and culture for the genetic counselling process.
- Identify and respond to the emerging needs of the client or family.
- Make a psychological assessment of the client's needs and resources and provide support, ensuring referral to other agencies as appropriate.
- Use a range of counselling skills to facilitate clients' adjustment and decision making.

Box 15.2 (Continued)

Management and organisation of care

- Document information including case notes and correspondence in appropriate manner.
- Identify, synthesise, organise and summarise relevant medical and genetic information for use in genetic counselling.
- Make appropriate and accurate genetic risk assessment.
- Identify and support clients' access to local, regional and national resources and services.
- Demonstrate ability to organise and prioritise a case load.

Professional and ethical practice

- Plan, organise and deliver professional and public education.
- Establish effective working relationships to function within a multidisciplinary team and as part of the wider health and social care network.
- Practice in accordance with the AGNC Code of Ethical Conduct.
- Recognise and maintain professional boundaries.
- Recognise his or her own limitations in knowledge and capabilities and discuss with colleagues or refer clients when necessary.
- Demonstrate reflective skills within the counselling context and in personal awareness for the safety of clients and families by participation in counselling/clinical supervision.
- Present opportunities for clients to participate in research projects in a manner that facilitates informed choice.

Professional and personal development

- Demonstrate continuing professional development as an individual practitioner and for the development of the profession.
- Develop the necessary skills to critically analyse research findings to inform practice development.
- Contribute to the development and organisation of genetic services.

(Association of Genetic Nurses and Counsellors, 2000b)

REGISTRATION BOARD

The next requirement was for the AGNC membership to appoint a registration board, whose remit is to assess applications for both initial and continued registration, including any circumstance that might affect the fitness of an individual to practice.

The board consists of ten elected members: seven registered genetic counsellors who are members of the AGNC, a clinical geneticist, an academic and a lay member.

ELIGIBILITY TO REGISTER

Applicants are eligible to register if they fulfil the following criteria:

- Possession of an approved master's degree in genetic counselling

or

- Possession of a relevant first or master's degree (e.g. in nursing, biological or social sciences), appropriate professional qualification (e.g. nursing, midwifery or health visiting), a minimum of two years' post-registration experience in a health or social care setting and basic training in counselling skills of at least 120 hours

or

- A minimum of two years' full-time (or part-time equivalent) experience working as a genetic counsellor prior to the inception of the scheme on 1 July 2001.

Those eligible to register are required to develop and submit a competency-based professional portfolio of evidence and attend an interview. Further details of the registration process can be found on the AGNC web site, www.agnc.org.uk.

GENETIC COUNSELLOR TRAINING POSTS

In 2003, the government white paper 'Our Inheritance, Our Future: Realising the potential of genetics in the NHS' (Department of Health, 2003) resulted in the establishment of genetic counsellor training posts in approved genetic centres. Graduate nurses and those with a master's degree in genetic counselling can apply for posts that provide the practical training and experience required. During the 27 months of training (full-time or part-time equivalent), trainees are encouraged and supported as they develop the competency-based professional portfolio required for accreditation and eventual registration as a genetic counsellor.

CAREER DEVELOPMENT

While most experienced genetic counsellors work in either a generic or familial cancer-related role, some have individual roles in different fields. Examples include foetal medicine, pre-implantation genetic diagnosis, disease specific roles, family support and research.

Those genetic counsellors employed by or attached to regional genetic centres may adopt specialist roles, including:

- A district-based role in a specific locality, which may be a district general hospital or primary care trust, managing the workload of that area.
- Cancer genetics.
- Integrated working with other specialities, for example neurology, ophthalmology, cardiology and foetal medicine.
- Education.
- Management.
- Research.

IMPLICATIONS FOR OTHER HEALTH PROFESSIONALS

In recent years, many well-respected, senior genetic professionals, together with other health professionals and their professional bodies, have lobbied MPs and the government to promote recognition of the value of genetics services and secure increased funding. The aim has been to develop the specialist genetics service while at the same time promoting increased genetic knowledge, skills and provision throughout the NHS.

These efforts have resulted in the government white paper 'Our Inheritance, Our Future: Realising the potential of genetics in the NHS' (Department of Health, 2003). In this white paper, the government formally recognises the impact that advances in human genetics will have on healthcare. In particular, it identifies five main objectives, which are to:

- Strengthen specialist genetic services. These currently care for individuals and the families of individuals who have or might be at risk of having an inherited disorder.
- Build genetics into mainstream services. This reflects the polygenic (interaction of many genes) nature of many common diseases and the possibility of using genetic testing to identify disease predisposition and instigate suitable management options.
- Spread genetics knowledge across the NHS. While the health professional training curriculum includes limited teaching of genetics, this needs to be revised and expanded if patients are to benefit.
- Generate new knowledge and applications. The need for continued research into areas such as pharmacogenetics and gene therapies is recognised.
- Ensure public confidence. The public needs to have access to unbiased, non-sensational and realistic information about the benefits of genetic knowledge (Department of Health, 2003).

These aims have huge implications for the NHS and for the specialised genetics services, which will need to support both primary care and mainstream services.

The government therefore identifies a number of initiatives which will support development, only a few of which will be discussed here.

NHS GENETICS EDUCATION AND DEVELOPMENT CENTRE

This centre was established in 2004 to help integrate genetics into the education and training of health professionals. The centre is working with professionals from many different disciplines to establish the extent of their genetics knowledge and the training needs relevant to their clinical practice, and to collect and develop training resources to meet the identified needs in the most appropriate way. Resources for health professionals learning and teaching genetics are available from the centre's web site, www.geneticseducation.nhs.uk.

FIT FOR PRACTICE IN THE GENETICS ERA

This research was conducted by the Genomics Policy Unit of the University of Glamorgan, with the aim of identifying the skills nurses, midwives and health visitors require to provide high-quality care for their patients. The final report identified seven core competencies, which are described as:

- Identify clients who might benefit from genetic services and information.
- Appreciate the importance of sensitivity in tailoring genetic information and services to clients' culture, knowledge and language level.
- Uphold the rights of all clients to informed decision making and voluntary action.
- Demonstrate a knowledge and understanding of the role of genetic and other factors in maintaining health and in the manifestation, modification and prevention of disease expression, to underpin effective practice.
- Demonstrate a knowledge and understanding of the utility and limitations of genetic testing and information.
- Recognise the limitations of one's own genetic expertise.
- Obtain and communicate credible, current information about genetics, for self, clients and colleagues.

The challenge now will be to incorporate these into both pre and post-registration training and thus everyday practice (Genomics Policy Unit & Medical Genetics Service for Wales, 2003).

EDUCATION IN GENETICS FOR HEALTH PROFESSIONALS

In October 2001, the Wellcome Trust and the Department of Health jointly commissioned the Public Health Genetics Unit in Cambridge to develop a strategy for the development of education for all health professionals, including policy makers, commissioners and health service managers (Burton, 2003).

DEVELOPMENT PROJECTS

A considerable number of diverse individual projects have been funded by the Department of Health with the aim of promoting genetics in both primary care and other mainstream services, as well as improving information available to the lay public. They include:

- Genetic knowledge parks.
- Genetic reference laboratories.
- General practitioners with a specialist interest in using genetics to support primary care practitioners.
- Projects aimed at improving multidisciplinary working, for instance joint speciality/genetic roles.
- Service development and delivery initiatives aimed at delivering genetics services in mainstream medicine.

CHALLENGE OF THE FUTURE

It is acknowledged that advances in genetic knowledge and technology can hold much hope for the future in terms of recognition of disease predisposition and more effective targeting of resources. However, resources are finite and all primary care trusts are faced with trying to meet the current health needs of their populations. Planning and investing for the future within budgetary restraints is always going to be difficult.

POINTS FOR REFLECTION

- Genetic counsellors are recruited from varied backgrounds, such as nursing, science and social working, so bring a diverse range of experience to the practice and development of both the profession and the service.
- How might you promote improved understanding and knowledge of genetics in your own sphere of practice?
- What do you see as the major challenge presented by the 'genetics era' to your own clinical practice?
- What do you feel are the advantages of the close links between the clinical, service laboratory and university genetics departments? Are there any disadvantages?

REFERENCES

American Society of Human Genetics, Ad Hoc Committee on Genetic Counselling (1975) Genetic counselling. *Am J Hum Genet*, **27**, 240–2.
Association of Genetic Nurses and Counsellors (2000a) Code of ethics. Available at: www. agnc.org.uk.

Association of Genetic Nurses and Counsellors (2000b) Core competencies. Available at: www.agnc.org.uk.

Association of Genetic Nurses and Counsellors (2003) Registration plan for genetic counsellors. Available at: www.agnc.org.uk.

Association of Genetic Nurses and Counsellors (2004) Assessment requirements. Available at: www.agnc.org.uk.

Burton, H. (2003) *Addressing Genetics Delivering Health*, Cambridge Public Health Genetics Unit.

Department of Health (2003) *Our Inheritance, Our Future: Realising the potential of genetics in the NHS*, The Stationery Office, London.

Genomics Policy Unit, University of Glamorgan and Medical Genetics Service for Wales, University Hospital of Wales (2003) Fit for practice in the genetics era: Final report to the Department of Health NHS genetic team. Available at: www.geneticseducation.nhs.uk/downloads/FitforPractice_FinalReport.pdf.

Weetman, M. (2002) *BSHG Newsletter*, **20**, 11–12.

16 Here and Now: Integrating Current Possibilities into Patient Care

PETER FARNDON

In Chapter 1, we reviewed some of the scientific and clinical advances which have led to our being able to apply genetics in clinical practice. But large challenges remain. How can a health system ensure that patients benefit from the genetics advances currently available? How can we encourage professionals to 'think genetics' when appropriate? How are the ethical and social issues surrounding the application of genetics to be discussed, adapted into professional life and, if necessary, reflected in government legislation?

In addition to the advances described in Chapter 1, the sequence of the human genome is now available. There is an expectation that this will assist in finding genes, understanding the effects of human genetic variation on the maintenance of health and the aetiology of disease, predicting susceptibility to diseases so that surveillance and prevention can be instituted, and that it will result in new forms of targeted therapy. But will people want to know this information and how will they act on it? How do we prepare a health system to assess the clinical usefulness of and adopt into practice advances which have not yet been made?

This chapter first looks at where genetics knowledge, skills and attitudes may be useful in current practice and then considers some issues for future practice, including the potential for therapy targeted according to the genetic makeup of host or pathogen.

WHERE CAN GENETICS CONTRIBUTE TO PATIENT CARE PATHWAYS?

All health workers agree that it is important to translate the promise of genetics into practical applications for patient care.

One very practical illustration is the family with the inherited predisposition to cancer described in Chapter 1. What were the steps taken to give the family the information they needed?

Genetics in Practice: A clinical approach for healthcare practitioners   Edited by Jo Haydon
© 2007 John Wiley & Sons, Ltd

First the family came to medical attention – in this case by their being concerned about the number of people affected in their family. Information was collected and the relationships of the affected people were determined, and represented in a family pedigree. The mode of inheritance of the condition was recognised, assessments were made of the probability that certain people could have inherited the predisposition, and then appropriate tests were organised. The information was shared with other family members and professionals.

Although the family had a particular genetic condition, the steps in this pathway are broadly the same for all genetic conditions. Different health professionals in different specialities will be involved in different stages of the pathway. A health professional in any role can therefore ask, 'What do I need to know and do about genetics?'

The NHS National Genetics Education and Development Centre and Skills for Health worked with health workers from many disciplines to identify the steps relating to genetics which are common to such pathways, and these are listed below as broad competences. They are designed to assist in meeting the healthcare needs of an individual and their family, including surveillance for potential complications and offering genetic information where appropriate.

A healthcare professional should be able to carry out those steps in the following pathway that are appropriate to his or her role:

1. Understand genetics within your area of clinical practice.
2. Identify patients with or at risk of genetic conditions.
3. Gather multi-generational family history information.
4. Use multi-generational family history information to draw a pedigree.
5. Recognise a mode of inheritance in a family.
6. Assess genetic risk.
7. Refer individuals to specialist sources of assistance in meeting their healthcare needs.
8. Recognise the indications for and the implications of ordering a molecular genetic test.
9. Communicate genetic information to patients, families and healthcare staff.

Although specialists in genetics would be expected to be able to undertake all these steps, for most health workers only certain steps will be appropriate. For example, while steps 1–4, 7 and 9 are likely to be applicable to health workers in many different roles, steps 5, 6 and 8 may be applicable only for those who have received training in genetics for specific defined roles.

Common to all the steps is the need to ensure that any genetic information a health worker gives to patients or colleagues is within the limits of their role, responsibility, knowledge and experience, and within consent and confidentiality guidelines relating to genetics issues.

Understand Genetics Within Your Area of Clinical Practice

In any work with patients, it is important that a health worker recognises the limits of, and progresses, their understanding of the subject. In addition, for genetics, as the subject is developing so rapidly, it is important that a health worker appreciates the (perhaps changing) impact genetics has on their particular area of practice and makes sure that patients can benefit from current services.

Care will benefit if the health worker has a basic awareness of genetic conditions that may occur within their clinical area, a working knowledge of population groups most at risk of genetic conditions and an awareness of ethical issues associated with genetics. It will be important to know how and where to access accurate up-to-date genetic information – through colleagues, electronically and through specialist genetic centres.

Identify Patients With or at Risk of Genetic Conditions

It is important that a health worker is able to use knowledge of genetics and of symptoms and clinical signs of genetic disorders within their area of practice to identify patients with or at risk of a genetic condition. Surveillance can then be instituted for potential complications and the offer of genetic information made where appropriate.

Techniques for identifying patients with or at risk of a genetic condition include using combinations of:

- Diagnosis of a condition known to be genetic, either in the patient or a family member.
- Identifying that several people within a family have the same condition.
- Knowledge of the genetic component of clinical conditions.
- Screening programmes.

There will be particular clinical questions related to the identification of disorders in the health worker's area of practice.

Gather Multi-Generational Family History Information

To assist in making a genetic diagnosis, it is often useful to gather accurate information about the immediate and extended family. Family history information can be used to draw a pedigree, recognise inheritance patterns and identify and asses genetic risks.

Information is usually gathered by face-to-face contact, but other methods, including the patient completing a family history form, are also used. In certain clinical pathways, the collection of family history information can be undertaken by non-clinical healthcare workers.

It is important to ask how people are related to each other, noting blood relatives, non-blood relatives and relatives from second or successive partnerships.

As well as recording living family members, it is important to note pregnancy losses, deaths (and their causes) and medical conditions within the family, and whether there are any particular environmental and lifestyle factors to which family members are exposed (see Chapter 2).

Use Multi-Generational Family History Information to Draw a Pedigree

Family history information can be presented as free text or in tables, but there is international recognition that the quickest and easiest way to record such information is to draw it graphically in the form of a pedigree, using standard symbols. This allows relationships and other information about a family to be seen at a glance (see Chapter 2).

Recognise a Mode of Inheritance in a Family

Disorders which appear to run in families may be caused by genetic factors, environmental influences or a combination of these. It is important to determine which of these is most likely to be the underlying cause as they may have different implications for other family members. It may be possible to be certain about the genetic basis for a condition when it is known to have a specific mode of inheritance, or when the pattern of affected people in the family fits with a pattern characteristic of a particular mode of inheritance. Some conditions (such as retinitis pigmentosa) can be inherited in several ways, and the pattern of affected members may provide the clue as to which mode of inheritance applies in a particular family (see Chapter 2). It is important to recognise the most likely basis for a condition so that the probabilities of being affected or of being carriers can be determined for other family members.

It is likely that health workers who need to make decisions about the mode of inheritance operating in particular families will have received appropriate genetics training.

Assess Genetic Risk

Assessment of genetic risk is usually undertaken in order to answer an individual's question about the likelihood of their having or being a carrier of a genetic condition, or of their having a baby with a genetic condition.

In some cases, for instance antenatal screening, a laboratory will provide a risk with its report which has been calculated through an algorithm or empiric risk tables. The health worker, having received training in the interpretation and explanation of this risk, will discuss it with the patient. In other cases, such as when risk has to be determined from a combination of a known diagnosis and family history information, risk assessment is best undertaken by healthcare workers who have received appropriate genetics training for specific defined roles. Where genetic risk assessment is required in situations which fall outside clinical protocols for non-genetics services, the patient should be referred to the specialist regional genetics service (see Chapter 5).

Refer Individuals to Specialist Sources of Assistance in Meeting Their HealthCare Needs

Although this step is an integral part of the genetics care pathway, it is, of course, common to all healthcare. The specific needs of a patient with a genetic disorder may require referral for surveillance, treatment or management of the disorder, or to specialist genetics services for risk assessment, genetic testing or to assist in family studies.

Recognise the Indications for and the Implications of Ordering a Molecular Genetic Test

Increasing numbers of genetic tests are becoming available. At present, nearly all are to detect disease-causing mutations for serious disorders inherited as single gene conditions. In the future, tests may be developed to look at multiple gene variants which, in particular combinations, predict the likelihood of an individual being affected by conditions such as diabetes or hypertension.

It is important when using genetic testing that a result will assist a specifically identified aspect of management. It may not be clinically necessary to offer a genetic test to every patient with a given condition. The clinical utility and validity of a particular genetic test needs to be agreed before it is accepted into a service such as the NHS. This is something that the Gene Dossier process of the UKGTN is designed to achieve – specific information about the patient population, the indications for the test, and the laboratory techniques are all assessed.

It is worth mentioning that, as well as from genetic laboratory testing, genetic information can be obtained from clinical examination, imaging and family history. For instance, a renal ultrasound scan in persons at risk of adult poly-cystic kidney disease could be defined as a genetic test in that it gives genetic information.

Once a genetic laboratory test is recognised as being appropriate for service, health workers need to bear in mind that the reason for ordering a genetic laboratory test is to inform clinical management and that the results may have implications for the patient and their family members.

A genetic test should usually be ordered by a healthcare worker in a specific defined role who has received appropriate genetics training, but most health workers would benefit from a broad understanding of when it might be appropriate to consider genetic testing.

Molecular genetic testing is used for:

- Diagnosis.
- Predictive testing.
- Testing for carrier status.
- Screening.
- Prenatal diagnosis.
- Pharmacogenetic testing (predicting response to therapy) (see Chapter 5).

Communicate Genetic Information to Patients, Family and HealthCare Staff

Usually a little extra time will be required to explain genetic information if the concepts of inheritance are not familiar to a patient. Some languages do not have specific words for genetic terms. The needs of the patient, including preferred language and method of communication, will need to be identified, and any translation service provided. A basic tenet of giving genetic information is that it should be presented in an understandable, non-directive manner, and the health worker should be aware of the impact genetic information may have on an individual or their family. It is important to agree with the patient on which other healthcare staff and family members may have access to their genetic information.

COMPETENCE FRAMEWORKS

The steps outlined above form the basis of a competence framework for non-genetics health workers and were designed by NHS staff, but they are likely to be transferable to other health and education systems. As stated above, in practice some competences will be applicable to a wide variety of health workers, while others will be relevant only to a small number of specialist healthcare professionals. They may be helpful in informing the development of job roles. Not all nine genetics competences will be applicable to every role; although the competences cover the whole of the pathway for a patient with, or at risk of, a genetic disorder, for any individual health professional only those genetic competencies relevant their agreed professional role to should be selected and included in a job description. These competences give an overview; specific details (e.g. which genetic conditions, which pathway) need to be determined locally.

Agreed competences can be used by individuals to develop their own knowledge, skills and performance; by education and training providers to identify learning needs, define learning outcomes and specify qualifications; and by organisations to set standards and improve the quality of services they offer. Support will be available from the NHS National Genetics Education and Development Centre (www.geneticseducation.nhs.uk).

Other competence frameworks have also been developed: for instance, the NCHPEG (National Coalition for Health Professional Education in Genetics) in the US has produced a comprehensive set of 35 competences for all health workers. The NCHPEG competences suggest that, as a minimum, each healthcare professional be able to:

- Appreciate limitations of his or her genetics expertise.
- Understand the social and psychological implications of genetic services.
- Know how and when to make a referral to a genetics professional.

The NCHPEG competences were adapted in the UK specifically for nursing, midwifery and health visiting professionals. They form a framework of seven competency statements, building on the general competences of a nursing role in the UK. They have been endorsed by the Nursing and Midwifery Council.

1. Identify clients who might benefit from genetic services and information through an understanding of the importance of family history in assessing predisposition to disease.
2. Appreciate the importance of sensitivity in tailoring genetics information and services to clients' culture, knowledge and language level.
3. Uphold the rights of all clients to informed decision making and voluntary action.
4. Demonstrate a knowledge and understanding of the role of genetics and other factors in maintaining health and in the manifestation, modification and prevention of disease expression, to underpin effective practice.
5. Demonstrate a knowledge and understanding of the utility and limitations of genetic testing and information.
6. Recognise the limitations of one's own genetics expertise.
7. Obtain and communicate credible, current information about genetics, for self, clients and colleagues.

These seven competency statements and the competences based on the patient pathway described above encompass the same basic concepts and map directly against one another.

ISSUES FOR FUTURE PRACTICE

This book has emphasised the practical aspects of genetics which a healthcare worker can use in their daily practice. However, much research is still needed to generate genetic advances that can be translated into clinically useful interventions or information. In addition, the adoption of genetic advances into clinical care needs to be supported by a framework of policies – not only in health but in other areas too, such as education, employment, insurance and protection of privacy. In addition, development of clinical services requires funding mechanisms to be identified, ideally in parallel with a system assessing the clinical utility of proposed advances.

First let us consider the major research effort to determine the human genome sequence, and then the policies needed to put new advances into clinical care.

WHAT WAS THE HUMAN GENOME PROJECT AND WHAT WILL IT OFFER?

The human genome project set out to discover all the estimated 20,000–25,000 human genes and to read and record the sequence of the 3,000,000,000 DNA subunits (bases) in the human genome. An integral part of the human genome project was to consider and address potential ethical, legal and social implications arising from project data. Researchers also studied the genetic makeup of several non-human organisms to help develop the technology and interpret human gene function by comparison across species. Organisms studied included the common human gut bacterium escherichia coli, the fruit fly, and the laboratory mouse.

There were major challenges. For instance, reading the human genome at a rate of one letter per second would take 31 years, reading continuously day and night.

At least 18 countries and 1000 researchers were involved in the public-sector human genome project, which the Human Genome Organisation (HUGO) helped to co-ordinate. The project began formally in October 1990 and was completed two years ahead of schedule, in 2003. There was a parallel private-sector project.

The human genome sequences published by both the international collaboration and the private-sector project do not represent any one person's genome, because DNA samples were anonymised and pooled for analysis. The private-sector project included anonymous donors of European, African, American (North, Central, South) and Asian ancestry. The leader of that project, Craig Venter, has since revealed that his own DNA sample was one of those in the pool.

In December 1999, the sequencing of the 33,400,000 base pairs of chromosome 22, containing at least 545 genes, was completed. Chromosome 21 followed in May 2000 – 33,500,000 base pairs but less than 300 genes.

Some companies and researchers decided to patent gene sequences. While patenting of an inventive step in designing a new technology has widespread support, many believed that the sequence of human genes should not be patented. The British Society for Human Genetics said: 'A natural gene sequence is not an invention, but is a discovered product of nature'. In March 2000, US President Bill Clinton and UK Prime Minister Tony Blair reaffirmed the international consortium's view that the raw sequence data should be freely available. This, they hoped, would encourage private investment in gene-based technologies, translating fundamental knowledge into medicinal products as quickly as possible.

Knowledge of the sequence of the human genome is already having an impact on the discovery of major genes associated with disease. A number of genes have been linked with breast cancer, muscle disease, deafness and blindness. In addition, understanding of the variation in the sequence between individuals, down to the level of single base changes (single nucleotide polymorphisms or SNPs) will be increasingly useful in determining which patterns of these changes are associated with the predisposition to such common diseases as cardiovascular disease, diabetes, arthritis and cancers, and with response to medical treatments.

HOW WILL UNDERSTANDING HUMAN GENETIC VARIABILITY BE USEFUL CLINICALLY?

It will be important to collect data on the usefulness of SNPs and other biomarkers in predicting disease susceptibility and response to treatments. UK Biobank is a medical research study of the impact on health of lifestyle, environment and genes in 500,000 people aged 40–69. Each participant donates blood and urine samples, has some standard measurements (such as blood pressure) and completes a confidential lifestyle questionnaire. Followed through the medical records of the NHS, over the next few decades the study will show the progression of illnesses such as cancer, heart disease, diabetes and Alzheimer's disease and will allow researchers to match these against genetic markers in the hope of developing new and better methods of prevention, diagnosis and treatment.

Already there are examples of how understanding a person's genetic makeup can impact on treatment options.

PHARMACOGENETIC DRUGS AND GENE-BASED DIAGNOSTIC TESTS

It is anticipated that for some treatments, the genetic makeup of the patient will be determined so that a drug or dose that is appropriate for the metabolism of that patient can be prescribed. It is already possible to test for genetic variants associated with the metabolism of warfarin, but the information on how to tailor the dose will not be available for routine clinical use until the results of clinical trials are known.

Crohn's disease is caused by environmental factors acting together with a complex genetic predisposition. Three variants in the CARD15 gene are strongly associated with Crohn's disease susceptibility and explain up to 20% of the genetic predisposition, but at present testing for them would not have a major impact on clinical practice. However, testing for variants in thiopurine methyltransferase (TPMT), which metabolises azathioprine (a mainstay of therapy in Crohn's disease), can determine the 10% of people with reduced activity of this enzyme, which results in adverse effects from the drug. In some healthcare systems, genetic screening is used to identify patients who will not tolerate a standard dose of the drug; in others, the dose of azathioprine is titrated clinically against side effects. But how will we be able to decide whether or not such testing should be clinically mandatory? We will need the information collected in clinical trials, and then a system to determine whether the test is appropriate to adopt into clinical practice.

Some drugs are being developed which specifically target the molecules made by certain types of tumours. To use these drugs, it will be the genetic constitution of the tumour, rather than the person, that must be determined. Herceptin and glivec are examples of targeted drugs which alter or block some very specific enzymes and receptors that lead to disease, and tend not to have the intolerable side effects of some of the non-specific cytotoxic drugs. Trastuzumab (herceptin) is an antibody for the treatment of breast cancer patients whose tumours overexpress HER-2, a growth factor receptor. Unless the patient's tumour overexpresses HER-2, treatment with this antibody drug is not effective – this is an example of determining the altered genetic constitution of a tumour, rather than looking for variations in the genes of a person.

Chronic myelogenous leukaemia is a cancer caused by a chromosomal rearrangement between two chromosomes resulting in a new gene product being formed which causes uncontrolled cell growth. Imatinib (glivec) is a small molecule which specifically inhibits the activity of this gene product and has a clinical response as high as 90%.

A NEED FOR SUPPORT THROUGH NATIONAL POLICIES

Exciting though advances in our understanding of genetic science are, translating these into practical clinical care needs a supportive policy environment.

The United Kingdom is fortunate in having a network of regional genetics services whose members are active in continually developing services and sharing best practice – for instance, the professional codes of confidentiality and consent in genetic practice proposed by the Joint Committee on Medical Genetics.

In addition, national bodies are actively involved in stimulating debate and developing and supporting policy. Bodies such as the Human Genetics Commission and the Nuffield Council on Bioethics are keeping a watching brief on genetics topics. The Human Genetics Commission (HGC), created by the government in 1999, provides strategic advice on human genetics, particularly on social, ethical and legal issues. It has considered genetics and reproductive decision-making; profiling babies at birth; storage, protection and use of personal genetic information; and genetic tests supplied directly to the public. The Gene Therapy Advisory Committee considers proposals for gene therapy research on human subjects. The Human Fertilisation and Embryology Authority is an independent regulator overseeing practice in fertility treatment and embryo research in the UK.

Concerns that the results of genetic tests might be used by insurance companies to the detriment of the population are well understood by the Department of Health's Genetics and Insurance Committee (GAIC). In October 2000, the committee agreed to allow insurers in the UK to use genetic test results in assessing the risk of Huntington disease. In 2005, the government and the insurance industry agreed on a 'Concordat and moratorium on genetics and insurance', which was informed by discussions between a wide range of interested parties.

In an attempt to ensure that molecular tests were available equitably to the UK population, the UK Genetic Testing Network was set up, and it now offers testing for 320 diseases. The UKGTN is a collaborative group of laboratories, clinicians and commissioners, and informed by patients. The UKGTN has developed a mechanism – the Gene Dossier process – for assessing the clinical usefulness of genetic tests before recommending that they are added to the portfolio of tests available through NHS funding. The process takes into account the seriousness and prevalence of the particular condition in a defined group of patients, the purpose, sensitivity, specificity, predictive value and cost of the test, and ethical, legal and social considerations. The UKGTN makes its recommendations on the timely introduction of new molecular testing to the Genetics Commissioning Advisory Group, which was set up by the Department of Health to take a strategic national overview of genetics in healthcare delivery. It aims to provide advice to commissioners of genetics services in order to enable them to provide appropriate services for NHS patients and their families.

In fact, the UK government has been taking an active interest in the potential for genetics to assist in tailoring medical interventions to prevent and treat according to need, as assessed by a person's genome. The Rt Hon. Alan Milburn MP, former Secretary of State for Health, instituted several initiatives. In January 2002 he explained the government's view on how the potential of genetics and the values of the NHS could work together:

> The values of Britain's National Health Service mean citizens can choose to take genetic tests free from the fear that should they test positive they face an enormous bill for insurance or treatment or become priced out of care or cover altogether. Properly exploited, genetics strengthens the case for the values of the NHS.

This optimistic view was not shared by several other governments, which were concerned that the 'genetics revolution' would place very high costs on health services – for genetic testing, for instance.

Alan Milburn also set up Genetics Knowledge Parks to try to encourage information resulting from the human genome project to be taken into patient care. A government white paper was published in 2003 and expanded previous government initiatives, setting up research projects in pharmacogenetics, gene therapy for cystic fibrosis and development of clinical and laboratory specialist services for genetics. As education had been highlighted in national reports as a key requirement for ensuring that the advances of genetics were given the highest chance of making an impact in clinical care, a national genetics education and development centre was established. The centre has been actively consulting many different healthcare groups to identify the core concepts in genetics which under-graduate training should cover. These should give a healthcare practitioner a mind map on which to pin new knowledge. The centre has also developed learning outcomes for undergraduate and postgraduate training, and workforce competences for practical application in patient care.

POINTS FOR REFLECTION

- Genetics is useful in clinical practice, making it important that every healthcare professional recognises the contribution that is appropriate to their role.
- There are is a prospect of real advances in clinical management in the future, particularly in design of drugs and understanding of how diseases such as cancer work.
- It is very important to have a continuum of genetics education, starting with basic concepts at undergraduate level and progressing to just-in-time information for clinical practice.

Glossary

Allele   Different forms of a gene found at a particular position on a chromosome.

Alpha-fetaprotein test (AFP)   A prenatal test to measure the amount of a foetal protein in the mother's blood. Abnormal amounts of the protein may indicate genetic problems in the foetus.

Amino acids   Chemical building blocks used to make proteins.

Amniocentesis   A prenatal test in which amniotic fluid containing foetal cells is withdrawn from the uterus, via the abdomen, for genetic or biochemical studies.

Aneuploidy   Having too few or too many copies of chromosomes. The common forms of aneuploidy in humans are trisomy (the presence of an extra chromosome) and monosomy (the absence of a single chromosome).

Anticipation   The tendency of some genetic conditions to increase in severity or appear earlier in successive generations of the same family.

Artificial insemination   The injection of semen into a woman's uterus (not through sexual intercourse) in order to make her pregnant.

Autosome   Any chromosome other than the sex chromosomes X and Y; 22 pairs in the human karyotype.

Banding   A technique of staining chromosomes in a characteristic pattern of lateral bands.

Bases   Distinct chemical ingredients found in the genetic material of all life-forms.

Base pair   Chemicals that pair to form DNA. Adenine (A) pairs with thymine (T); cytosine (C) pairs with guanine (G).

Bias of ascertainment   Distortions in a set of data caused by the way cases are collected, for example, severely affected people are more likely to be recognised than mildly affected people.

Carrier   A healthy person who has one normal gene and one altered gene for a recessively inherited disease, or a person with a balanced chromosome rearrangement. In either case, the carrier has a normal phenotype.

Centromere   The primary constriction of the chromosome, separating it into its two arms. It is attached to the spindle fibres at mitosis and meiosis.

Chorionic villus sampling (CVS)   A prenatal test in which a few milligrams of placental tissue (chorionic villi) are removed (vaginally or abdominally). The tissue is then used to examine the chromosomes or perform DNA tests.

Genetics in Practice: A clinical approach for healthcare practitioners   Edited by Jo Haydon
© 2007 John Wiley & Sons, Ltd

Chromosome Rod-like structures that carry the genes, consisting of long strands of DNA in a protein framework. In non-dividing cells they are not individually distinguishable in the nucleus, but at mitosis or meiosis they become condensed into visible strands that stain deeply with basic stains.

Chromosome painting Fluorescence labelling of a whole chromosome by a FISH procedure in which the probe is a cocktail of many different DNA sequences from a single chromosome.

Clinical genetics The branch of genetics concerned with the diagnosis of genetic conditions and genetic counselling for families.

Clone To make an exact copy of.

Coding sequence The sequence of bases in DNA which specifies the structure of a protein.

Congenital Present at birth; may or may not have a genetic cause.

Consanguineous Refers to a mating between two people who are related by blood (i.e. share one common ancestor).

Consultand The individual (not always affected) referred for genetic counselling.

Cordocentesis A prenatal test in which a foetal blood sample is obtained from the umbilical cord. This may also be referred to as foetal blood sampling (FBS).

Cytogenetics The branch of genetics concerned with the physical structure and appearance of chromosomes.

Cytoplasm The jelly-like material which surrounds a cell's nucleus.

Deletion The loss of a segment of DNA from a chromosome. It may be of any length, from a single base to a large part of the chromosome.

Diploid Having two copies of each chromosome; the normal constitution of most human somatic cells.

DNA (deoxyribonucleic acid) The substance that contains genetic material, found in chromosomes in the cell nucleus. The genetic instructions contained in DNA are needed to build a living being and for the day to day activities of each body cell.

Dominant A characteristic that is apparent when there is only one copy of the particular gene present, or in the case of a genetic disease when only one copy is altered.

Dysmorphic The unusual or abnormal appearance of one or more parts of the body.

Dysmorphology The clinical study of malformation syndromes.

Empiric risk Risk estimate based on experience rather than calculation.

Exon A segment of a gene that is represented in the mature RNA product. Individual exons may contain coding DNA and/or non-coding DNA.

Expressivity Extent to which a gene is clinically evident (expressed) in an individual.

Familial A trait that occurs more often in the relatives of an affected person than in the general population, e.g. diabetes, coronary heart disease.

FISH Fluorescence *in situ* hybridisation is a laboratory technique that uses a fluorescently labelled DNA or RNA probe to detect subtle changes in the chromosome structure.

Founder effect High frequency of a particular allele in a population due to that population being derived from a small number of founders, one or more of whom carried that allele.

Gamete A germ cell formed in the reproductive organs; a sperm or ovum.

Gene   The unit of inheritance, consisting of a sequence of DNA.

Gene dosage   The number of copies of a gene. Abnormal dosage of some genes (e.g. trisomy) can cause developmental abnormalities.

Gene variant   A difference in the DNA sequence of a gene from the usual sequence. Most gene variants are harmless but some can cause a genetic disorder.

Gene tracking   Following a gene through a family by observing the inheritance of a marker that is inherited alongside the gene.

Genetic counselling   A communication process intended to help an individual or family understand a condition, assist in decision making and offer support.

Genome   All the genes present on a set of chromosomes.

Genotype   The genetic constitution of an individual.

Gonadal mosaicism   Presence of a mutation in germline but not somatic cells, which results in transmission of a genetic disorder by a healthy person.

Haploid   The normal number of chromosomes present in an egg or sperm. In humans, the haploid number of chromosomes is 23.

Hemizygous   Having only one copy of a gene or DNA sequence in diploid cells. Males are hemizygous for most genes on the sex chromosomes. Deletions occurring on one autosome produce hemizygosity in males and females.

Heterogeneity   The phenomenon by which a certain phenotype (or clinical feature) can be produced by different genetic mechanisms.

Heterozygote   An individual having different forms of a gene (allele) at a certain position on a pair of chromosomes.

Homologous   A pair of chromosomes carrying the same genes in the same order.

Homozygote   An individual having two identical forms of a gene (allele) at a certain position on a pair of chromosomes.

Imprinting   Determination of the expression of a gene by its parental origin.

Index case   The individual who is first referred to the geneticist.

Insertion   The addition of a segment of DNA, which may be of any length.

Intron   Non-coding (nonsense) DNA, which separates exons in a gene.

Inversion   The alteration in a sequence of genes within a chromosome. In a paracentric inversion the change occurs on one side of the centromere. In a pericentric inversion the centromere is involved.

Karyotype   The classified chromosome complement of an individual or cell.

Linkage   The tendency of genes or other DNA sequences at specific loci to be inherited together as a consequence of their physical proximity on a single chromosome.

Locus   The precise location of a gene or DNA marker on a chromosome.

Marker   Biochemical or DNA polymorphism occurring close to a gene and used in gene tracking.

Meiosis   The production of gametes.

Mendelian disorder   Inherited disorder due to a defect in a single gene.

Missense mutation   A nucleotide substitution that results in an amino acid change.

Mitochondria   Organelles in a cell's cytoplasm, chiefly responsible for energy production.

Mitochondrial inheritance   Transmission of a mitochondrial trait, exclusively through female relatives.

Mitosis   The production of somatic diploid cells.

Monosomic   Having only one of the genes, DNA segments or whole chromosomes from a pair of homologous chromosomes.

Mosaic   The presence of two or more cell lines which differ from each other in genotype or chromosome number.

Multifactorial   Inheritance due to the interaction between a number of genes and environmental factors.

Mutation   A permanent change or alteration in the structure of DNA.

Non-disjunction   Failure of paired chromosomes to separate during cell division; the major cause of numerical chromosome abnormalities.

Non-penetrance   A genetic mutation that does not cause a genetic condition to occur, due to the effect of other genetic loci or of the environment.

Pedigree   A graphic representation of a person's family, also known as a family tree.

Penetrance   Likelihood that a genetic mutation will cause a genetic condition to occur.

Phenotype   The observable or clinical characteristics of an individual.

Polymorphism   The existence of genes at a particular position on a chromosome with an altered DNA sequence, usually non-pathological.

Prenatal diagnosis   A test done on a foetus during pregnancy to determine whether it has a particular disorder.

Proband   The individual who draws medical attention to a family.

Recessive   A characteristic that is only apparent when there are two copies of a particular gene present, one from each parent.

Reciprocal translocation   A chromosomal rearrangement involving exchange of chromosome material between at least two chromosomes.

Recurrence risk   The probability that a genetic condition will occur again.

Robertsonian translocation   A chromosomal rearrangement that converts two acrocentric chromosomes into one metacentric.

Segregation ratio   The proportion of offspring who inherit a given gene or character from a parent.

Sex chromosomes   The chromosomes responsible for sex determination (XX in women; XY in men).

Sex-linked   Inheritance of a gene carried on a sex chromosome.

Siblings/sibs   A person's brothers and sisters.

Single gene disorder   A disease whose inheritance is controlled by one pair of genes (one on each homologous chromosome).

Somatic cell   Any cell in the body except the eggs or sperm.

Somatic mutation   A gene fault that occurs after fertilisation and is found only in cells that are derived from the originally mutated cell.

Southern blot   Laboratory technique for analysing DNA.

Stem cells   Type of cell that has the ability to produce unlimited numbers of either new stem cells or daughter cells, which will become specialised to perform a certain function.

Syndrome   A collection of physical findings that occur together frequently enough to be recognised as a distinct clinical entity.

Telomere   A specialised structure at the tip of chromosomes. It consists of an array of short tandem repeats, TTAGGG in humans, which form a closed loop and protect the chromosome end.

Teratogen   An agent capable of causing congenital malformations, e.g. drugs, radiation.

Trait   Any gene-determined characteristic.

Translocation   The transfer of chromosomal material between chromosomes.

Triplet repeat   A sequence of three bases that is repeated more than once within a gene.

Trisomy   Three copies of a given chromosome per cell.

Tumour suppressor gene   A gene that prevents abnormal growth of cells.

Uniparental disomy   A cell in which both copies of one particular chromosome pair are derived from one parent, with no contribution from the other parent. This may or may not be pathogenic, depending on the chromosome involved.

Variable expression   Variation in the severity of symptoms in a genetic disorder in different individuals.

X-inactivation (lyonisation)   The early inactivation of one of the two X chromosomes in females, allowing expression of genes on the active X chromosome only.

X-linked   Genes carried on the X chromosome.

Zygote   The fertilised egg cell.

Useful Websites

Antenatal Results and Choices
www.arc-uk.org

Antenatal Screening Web Resource (AnSWeR)
www.antenataltesting.info

Association of Genetic Nurses and Counsellors
www.agnc.org.uk

Bowel Cancer UK
www.bowelcanceruk.org.uk

Breast Cancer Care
www.breastcancercare.org.uk

British Society for Human Genetics
www.bshg.org.uk

Cancerbackup
www.cancerbackup.org.uk

Cancer Research UK
www.crc.org.uk

Contact-a-Family (umbrella-group listing of many UK support groups for families with disabled children)
www.cafamily.org.uk

DIPEx (personal experiences of health and illness)
www.dipex.org

Fit for Practice in the Genetic Era
www.geneticseducation.nhs.uk/downloads/FitforPractice_Extendedsummary.pdf

Nursing Standard (series of seven articles about genetic competences)
www.nursing-standard.co.uk/professionaldevelopment/genetics.asp

Genetics Interest Group (national organisation representing over 120 charities supporting children, families and individuals affected by genetic disorders)
www.gig.org.uk

Genetics in Practice: A clinical approach for healthcare practitioners Edited by Jo Haydon
© 2007 John Wiley & Sons, Ltd

GeneTests (clinical information resource)
www.genetests.org

International Society of Nurses in Genetics (ISONG)
www.isong.org

National Coalition for Health Professional Education in Genetics (NCHPEG)
www.nchpeg.org

National Genetics Education and Development Centre (NGEDC)
www.geneticseducation.nhs.uk

UK Newborn Screening Programme Centre
www.newbornscreening-bloodspot.org.uk

Nuffield Council on Bioethics
www.nuffieldbioethics.org

Ovacome (ovarian cancer support network)
www.ovacome.org.uk

PHG Foundation (news and information about advances in genetics, their impact on public health and the prevention of disease)
www.phgfoundation.org

UK Genethics Club (national forum for the discussion, by health professionals, of practical ethical problems arising in clinical genetics practice)
www.genethicsclub.org

Your Genes, Your Choices: Exploring the issues raised by genetic research
www.ornl.gov/hgmis/publicat/genechoice

Index